Veterinary Science: A Very Short Introduction

VERY SHORT INTRODUCTIONS are for anyone wanting a stimulating and accessible way into a new subject. They are written by experts, and have been translated into more than 45 different languages.

The series began in 1995, and now covers a wide variety of topics in every discipline. The VSI library currently contains over 550 volumes—a Very Short Introduction to everything from Psychology and Philosophy of Science to American History and Relativity—and continues to grow in every subject area.

Very Short Introductions available now:

Available soon:

For more information visit our website

www.oup.com/vsi/

James Yeates

VETERINARY SCIENCE

A Very Short Introduction

Great Clarendon Street, Oxford, OX2 6DP,
United Kingdom

Oxford University Press is a department of the University of Oxford.
It furthers the University's objective of excellence in research, scholarship,
and education by publishing worldwide. Oxford is a registered trade mark of
Oxford University Press in the UK and in certain other countries

Published in the United States of America by Oxford University Press
198 Madison Avenue, New York, NY 10016, United States of America

British Library Cataloguing in Publication Data

Data available

Library of Congress Control Number: 2017956922

ISBN 978-0-19-879096-9

Printed in Great Britain by
Ashford Colour Press Ltd, Gosport, Hampshire

Contents

List of illustrations

Prologue

If you want to know about veterinary science, this book is for you. Someone who cares about animals, anyone who cares about human health, and everyone who cares about the environment needs to understand the connections between humans' and other animals' health and welfare. Veterinary medicine is all about the interactions of people, animals, and the environment.

I was extremely excited when asked to write this book. The VSI series has helped me learn more about many fields outside and within my own expertise, and this book can help others to gain the same insights about veterinary science. This book takes readers through key tenets, principles, controversies, challenges, and future directions. It highlights topical and current 'big issues' across the globe, and across all aspects of veterinary science.

Veterinary science is in the middle of the hourglass between our past and our future. Five millennia of veterinary science have forged our ability to help a wide range of animals. The next five decades are expected to bring rapid, global changes and we will need veterinary science to meet the challenges, and embrace the opportunities, of this future. Key to this will be its role in achieving ambitious economic, public health, social, and environmental goals.

The future will need greater collaboration across traditional fields, reforming the links that specialization has strained. So I have tried to encompass all science concerned with animals' bodily and mental health, knowing that many of the researchers in these areas might not have previously thought of themselves as contributing to veterinary science. It is only by fully understanding one another that we can ensure our collective actions will help and protect animals and, by doing so, help and protect ourselves. And I hope that this book provides even a tiny bit of the inspiration that other VSIs have given me.

My thanks to the many who have commented on drafts, in particular Heather Bacon, John Blackwell, David Burch, Andrew Butterworth, David Catlow, Simon Doherty, Andrew Gardiner, Peter Jinman, Robert Johnson, Paolo Martelli, Frank McMillan, Carla Molento, Alex Singleton, Sean Wensley, Abigail Woods, Julia Wrathall, anonymous external reviewers, and the editors.

Chapter 1
All creatures great and small

An ancient profession

Just as for our patients, understanding our profession's history—its 'genetics' and past behaviour—can help us work out what to do next in our future. This abridged history—the reality was doubtless much messier at the time—helps highlight important themes, in particular how veterinary scientific developments have come hand-in-paw with progress in other scientific fields, and alongside social changes in how we treat animals.

Caring for our animals' health and welfare probably goes back further than recorded human history. Prehistoric shepherds and farmers almost certainly treated their livestock and dogs for common injuries and diseases. They probably also shared microbes, such as the bacterial ancestor of the *Mycobacterium* that causes tuberculosis, and more beneficial gut bacteria. Within recorded history, looking back as far as we can, the oldest known person who can be described as a veterinary scientist is Urlugaledinna, who was an 'expert in healing animals' from around 3000 BC in Mesopotamia (Figure 1). Later, the laws of the Mesopotamian city Eshnunna (*c.*1930 BC) decreed that owners could be fined if people died after having been bitten by their dogs; more than a century later, the famous Babylonian Code of

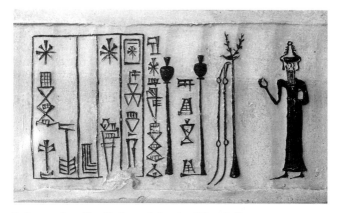

1. Impression of a cylinder seal showing Urlugaledinna.

Hammurabi (*c*.1754 BC) gave guidance to both veterinary and human physicians—including how to set professional fees.

Elsewhere, the Ancient Egyptians used herbal medicines for animals and aspects of veterinary science (particularly gynaecology) were recorded in the fragmentary Egyptian Kahun papyri (*c*.1825 BC). Further east, in India during the Vedic period (*c*.1500–*c*.500 BC), a famous healer named 'Salihotra' described how to treat—and prevent—various diseases of horses and elephants. Among other matters, he described a wide variety of horse types, including horses 'the colour of a conch shell' and 'having the smell of ghee'. Perhaps more significantly in scientific terms, he highlighted important medical conditions such as dental disease and emaciation. Since both horses and elephants were essential in Ancient India for transportation and war, protecting their health was of vital service to the Vedic civilization.

In Ancient China, legend has it that veterinary medicine had been begun by the Emperor Fuxi, and was progressed by the Chinese 'divine farmer' Shennong who wrote about drugs and described the disease that we now know as tuberculosis. Outside legend, there is evidence that the Western Zhou dynasty (1046–771 BC) had a veterinary department within its administration and the first records of a structured veterinary *profession* come from China in around 400 BC, where aspiring veterinarians had to sit entrance examinations that emphasized the importance of veterinary science in protecting the public's health.

Ancient Greek scientist-philosophers such as Democritus (*c.*460–c.370 BC) and Aristotle (384–322 BC) advanced the study of animals' bodies, using autopsies and vivisection, and noted that rabies (Box 1) could be spread by bites from 'irritable' dogs. Meanwhile, Hippocrates (*c.*460–c.375 BC) developed his theory of humours, which dominated medicine, including veterinary medicine, for the next 2,000 years. Aristotle's star pupil and eventual successor, Theophrastus (*c.*371–c.287 BC), wrote extensive works on botany (e.g. 'Enquiry into Plants'), human physiology (e.g. 'On Sweat, on Fatigue, on Dizziness') and various documents on other animals (e.g. 'On Fish'). In particular, Theophrastus added to Aristotle's studies on animals' bodies by investigating their environments, behaviour, and psychology, highlighting more similarities between humans and other species that led him to conclude that neither should be subjected to cruelty.

Box 1 Rabies

Lyssaviruses can spread to all mammals (especially bats, dogs, and other carnivores) and birds. Bites transmit the virus in the saliva, which travels slowly up the nerves to the brain, eventually (sometimes after many months) causing either nervousness or fearlessness, aggression, altered voices, mal-coordination, paralysis, and is almost certainly fatal if untreated. Prevention involves quarantine, human education to prevent dog bites or keeping wildlife as pets, and replacing inhumane culling with vaccination programmes.

Back in India, around 250 BC, the King Ashoka had edicts inscribed on pillars and rocks that protected a range of animals, including parrots, bats, terrapins, fish, squirrels, deer, bulls, and both wild and domestic pigeons. He forbade castrating cockerels or feeding one animal to another. His edicts stated that the King had provided for medical treatment for all, both human and other animals. King Ashoka also directed the growth and importation of medical herbs and roots to treat both humans and animals, and created large numbers of animal hospitals, although eventually these were largely destroyed by invasions.

A prominent Roman veterinary profession is found too, particularly looking after cattle ('*veterinae*' in Latin). Varro (116–27 BC) wrote about farming and the diseases such as malaria that were associated with swamps, and the Roman government appointed inspectors to check that market traders were selling healthy meat. Cardanus described rabid dogs' saliva as a poison ('*virus*' in Latin) and, in the 3rd century AD, Vegetius suggested cauterizing dog bites to prevent rabies—alongside applying dog-rose roots, putting patients in the dark so they cannot see water, and feeding them

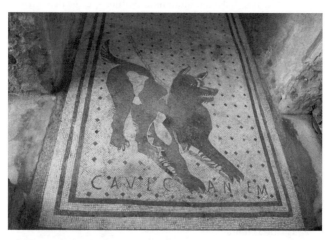

2. Cave canem: a Roman mosaic in Pompeii.

the boiled liver of the dog who bit them (Figure 2). The famous Galen (129–c. 200/216 AD) used farm animal dissection to develop the ideas that became the cornerstone of medicine. Vivisection was also popular in Roman times, but less as scientific endeavour as for public entertainment, alongside gladiatorial combat, executions, and animal fights.

Out of the darkness

As the Roman world shrunk into the Byzantine Empire, veterinary progress was limited. Nevertheless, Apsyrtus (the real person, not the mythological character), who accompanied the Emperor Constantine (c.272–337 AD) in his military expeditions, tried to make veterinary medicine more scientific, and suggested methods such as isolating ill individuals, splinting fractures, and stitching up wounds. His writings on the veterinary care of horses—important in Constantine's wars—were very practical guides after the humorous and malodorous theorizing in earlier works.

However, such progress was too limited to stop the bubonic plague (Box 2) that struck the Byzantine Empire in 541 AD. This disease killed large numbers of humans, although the Emperor Justinian managed to survive. It also decimated populations of other animals, including many wild animals that predators needed

Box 2 Bubonic plague

Yersinia pestis bacteria are spread by biting fleas across many species including rodents and humans. Infections can cause enlarged 'bubonic' lymph nodes, multi-organ infection or cough, and is often fatal if untreated (as often the case in remote areas). It continues to occur nowadays in Madagascar, the Democratic Republic of Congo, and Peru. Prevention involves preparing for outbreaks due to climate change, biological warfare, or drug-resistance.

to eat, thereby causing widespread disruption to the natural ecosystems. As veterinary science, like other sciences, dwindled during the dark ages, much of the surviving knowledge was maintained by Persian, Arabian, and Islamic authors. Such authors drew on Indian, Roman, and Byzantine texts, maintaining a focus on keeping horses healthy for transportation and war.

Animal diseases followed the Hun armies as they invaded Europe in the 5th century, and then the Crusaders as they travelled east six centuries later. Some new cures for animal disease were described in the Anglo-Saxon *Leech Book*, which was possibly written in the 9th century, under Alfred the Great. However, around the 11th century, a 'cattle plague' appeared, which was to cause untold misery for countless cows and farmers in the coming centuries. This now appears to be a viral disease related to measles (both viruses probably evolved from an earlier virus that is now extinct) but at the time, there seemed no reason for the widespread destruction.

Then, in the 14th century, the bubonic plague struck Eurasia again, with catastrophic results: the 'Black Death'. The disease spread west, probably alongside severe weather, and widespread human cases were recorded by Arab writers, such as Ibn Al-Wardni and Almaqrizi, and by European novelists such as Boccaccio. Meanwhile, rabid dogs were not only a health risk to the general public and other animals, but became a common theme for medieval moral and political works—whose authors drew metaphors from the observation that dogs sometimes return to eat their own vomit.

After the Reconquista ended in 1492, the new Catholic Spanish monarchs patronized horse healers known as *albeiteras*, and established the first real European veterinary schools, which sadly did not last. Across Europe, Roman and Greek works, such as Galen's and Vegetius's, were still well-thumbed and commonly printed on the new presses, but contemporary writers also began to add to the science. In England, Thomas Blundeville wrote *The fower chiefyst offices belonging to horsemanshippe* in 1565, which he promised would help the gentlemen of England to 'passe the Frenchmen and all other nations'. In Italy, Carlo Ruini wrote his *Anatomia del cavallo, infermita, et suoi rimedii*, which was published in 1598, dividing horses' anatomy into 'soulful', 'spiritual', 'nutritive', 'generative', and skeletal parts. Meanwhile, colonizing conquistadores spread a variety of diseases to South America, including smallpox.

The Roman Catholic Church was by no means as opposed to scientific progress as is often alleged, although the dissection of human bodies was officially forbidden. Instead, pigs were used to teach both swine and human anatomy in medical schools such as Salerno and Padua. The animals were generally dissected while they were still *alive* and without anaesthetic. In a famous contemporaneous report, one student at Padua pulled a puppy from the womb of a vivisected bitch. When he hurt the puppy, she barked at him; when he raised the puppy to her mouth, she licked her offspring. Watchers were interested in this example of maternal love in a 'brute'. The use of non-human animals in medical education helped to establish the importance of comparative medicine as a central part of both medical and veterinary sciences, which would later lead to the conclusions that such studies are ethically unacceptable.

Enlightened veterinarians

Veterinary science, like so many other scientific studies, began to resemble the modern field of today during the scientific revolution from the 17th century, and the Enlightenment of the 18th century. European scientists learnt about physiology by dissecting—and vivisecting—animals. For the latter purposes, the scientists often used dogs because they tended to be more compliant, but they dissected a wide range of species, including human criminals and mental health patients. Public animal experimentation also became a popular entertainment again. Famous scientists such as Robert Boyle and John Hooke used vacuums to show members of the Royal Society in London that a dazzling range of species die without oxygen.

The work of surgeons like John Hunter showed yet more similarities between animal species. But some of these Enlightenment scientists argued that non-human animals, contrary to all appearances, were unable to feel pain. This view certainly helped them to defend their practice against challenges such as the poet Alexander Pope's question to his friend, the scientist Stephen Hales who was best known for his work on blood pressure, 'How do we know that we have a right to kill creatures that we are so little above as dogs?' Many other scientists did recognize that animals could feel pain, including the naturalist John Ray. Meanwhile, Christian groups began to re-affirm the wrongness of animal cruelty, eventually leading to the formation of the Royal Society for the Prevention of Cruelty to Animals (RSPCA) in 1824 by a group including the anti-slavery campaigner William Wilberforce.

Back on the farm, there were still many diseases to overcome. Sheep began to suffer a new neurological disease that made many of them scratch their skin on fences and bushes, damaging their valuable wool—hence the name 'scrapie'. Ironically, it became more common as farmers in-bred certain bloodlines for better wool. Cows were still being killed by cattle plague, spread by armies such as Peter the Great's. Meanwhile, a closely related virus was spreading through Europe's dogs. The English claimed it came from France; the French claimed it came from England; a more recent theory suggests it came from South America—in exchange for European diseases like smallpox. This disease caused thickening of dogs' feet (hence the name 'hardpad'); coughing (hence another name, 'dog influenza'); white, flaky skin and neurological problems (hence 'distemper'). It probably killed one in every three ill dogs, and other dogs were probably killed because people thought they were rabid.

There was no cure for scrapie, cattle plague, or distemper. Several people ran distemper nursing homes, but euthanasia was often the treatment given for severe cases—although experiences from Asia suggest that, nowadays, good supportive therapy can help most patients recover. However, the diseases could be stopped from spreading. In 1711, Pope Clement XI asked the physician Giovanni Lancisi, who first made the link between malaria and mosquitoes, to study cattle plague. Lancisi recommended methods such as quarantine, pre-movement health certificates, and removing ill animals to stop the disease spreading. He also recommended that animal health be developed as a specialism within medicine. At the same time, in England, Thomas Bates developed other methods to control cattle plague, which were also effective but not widely applied.

Also in England, the surgeon-and-farrier William Gibson began to teach about humane and scientific treatments for animals. But it was in France, devastated by cattle plague and military horse losses, that the first modern veterinary school was created. A desperate French government turned to a wealthy nobleman Claude Bourgelat, who was the Director of the Lyon Academy of Equitation where young men were taught horse-riding, fencing, music, and etiquette. He was asked to establish a school 'to teach the knowledge and treatment of the diseases of all domestic animals' and, in 1762, he opened a school in a disused tavern for six students, with the entrance requirements of being (a) literate and (b) baptized. A second, Parisian school soon followed (whose students defended the town during the Franco-Prussian war) and nineteen more European veterinary schools were established that century including the London Veterinary College—compared to only six new facilities for treating human patients.

During the 18th century, there were significant developments in our understanding of microbes, how diseases are spread, and how our bodies can fight off these microbes. Of particular note is the work on helping patients to increase their immunity against particular germs. Several European scientists identified that previous infection with cowpox (*Vaccinia* in Latin) could provide human patients with some protection against smallpox. This observation eventually led to the development of an effective vaccine against smallpox, when an English scientist (Edward Jenner) vaccinated an 8-year-old boy (James Phipps) using cowpox viruses from a milkmaid (Sarah Nelmes) who had been infected by a cow (Blossom). Such efforts also helped to discredit the old medical ideas of humours, miasmas, and the theory that diseases could spontaneously generate from nothing.

A belle époque?

At the start of the 19th century, the German scientist, Georg Gottfried Zinke, demonstrated that rabies could be passed through saliva from rabid dogs. Through the century, various scientists including Jean-Joseph-Henri Toussaint, Louis Pasteur, and Robert Koch further explored and popularized the idea that diseases were spread by tiny 'germs', and created various vaccines against anthrax and rabies. Louis Pasteur and colleagues produced the latter by infecting rabbits, killing them, and drying out infected nerves to kill or weaken the virus, testing the resultant vaccine in dogs before giving it to a young boy who had been bitten by a rabid dog. Most famously, Pasteur helped to develop a method to kill off (most of) the bacteria in drinks—pasteurization—that is now used to remove tuberculosis and other microbes from milk.

The mid-19th century also saw the dissemination of many new developments in veterinary techniques (Figure 3). It also saw the budding of formal medical professions in the UK, with the creation of the Royal College of Veterinary Surgeons in 1844 and the General Medical Council a little later, in 1858. The same decades provided massive advances in our understanding. Rudolf Virchow convincingly discredited the ancient theory of humours, described the life-cycle of tapeworms (*Trichinella spiralis*), and developed methods of autopsy and meat inspections.

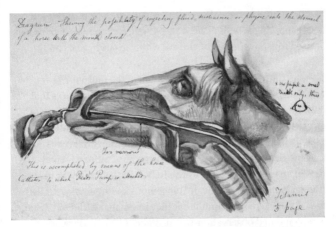

3. 'Watercolour diagram showing the possibility of injecting fluid sustenance or physic into the stomach of a horse with the mouth closed' by Edward Mayhew (1808–68).

Governments increasingly centralized the organization of slaughterhouses, so that hygiene and meat quality could be better checked and controlled. Meanwhile, the independent findings of Charles Darwin and the friar Gregor Mendel described how animals can inherit characteristics from their parents, and pass them onto their offspring, with some potential for changes across generations. This work also provided additional, if controversial, evidence for the genetic links between humans and other animals.

In the late 19th century, animal breeding created a variety of types, most notably of dogs, but also of 'fancy' mice, rats, birds, and cats. This was driven partly by human enjoyment of novelty or show success, partly through the snobbery of wanting 'purebred' animals, and perhaps partly by concern over diseases such as distemper found in mongrels on the street—although purebreds are not immune to such infections, as is sadly clear in modern puppy farms. Unfortunately, such breeds, through inbreeding and desires for particular body shapes and facial appearances, caused a similar variety of breed-related illnesses. Historically, animals had been bred to have the health needed for their purpose—ill dogs cannot fight bulls or herd sheep well. But animals kept as pets or used for showing might survive with various health conditions.

The end of the century saw the creation of the journal *The Veterinary Record*, whose first editorial advised its readers that 'we have too long accustomed ourselves to a respectful following of our sister profession [of medicine]'. This occurred just after, in 1881, British politicians brought in the Veterinary Surgeons Act that restricted the title 'veterinary surgeon' to those who had passed an examination set by the RCVS. In the same year in Russia, Ivan Pavlov and Ivan Tolochinov experimentally studied how dogs reacted to stimuli that they associated with food, which complemented observation-based studies (such as Darwin's) and helped us understand how animals actively respond and adapt to their environment. Meanwhile, to reduce some of these reactions, anaesthetics (discovered in the 1840s) began to be used more commonly to allow patients to be unconscious during surgery and some vivisection.

As the 19th century ended, the threats to animal health continued. Cattle plague was accidentally spread to Africa by European colonial soldiers, where it killed hundreds of millions of wild and domestic animals that had limited immunity to a European microbe. This devastation, combined with a concurrent drought, caused a severe famine that killed up to 75 per cent of the affected Maasai people of Kenya and Tanzania, and destroyed communities such as the Basotho people of southern Africa. In East Africa, during 1889–96, the combination of colonial expansion, cattle plague, and natural disasters deprived Tsetse flies of their food, making them turn to humans, spreading sleeping sickness (Box 3). In the mid-19th and early 20th century, another wave of bubonic plague spread across India and around the Pacific to Australia and Hawaii. In the USA, hog cholera (later called classical swine fever) affected thousands of pigs—and farmers. The veterinary scientist Dr Daniel Salmon discovered that some of these pigs also were

Box 3 Trypanosomiasis

Different species of Trypanosome microbes infect many different species, including cows, sheep, goats, dogs, and humans. They are spread by Tsetse flies and other biting flies. Various symptoms are caused by the patient's immune responses and can well be fatal if untreated. Several drugs may cure or prevent the disease but, because variations in the microbes makes creating a vaccine difficult, the key prevention methods aim at limiting the spread of the Tsetse fly, for example by releasing 'neutered' flies.

Box 4 Influenza

Various types of influenza viruses infect many species, including pigs, horses, ducks, and ferrets. Many forms cause few problems in their usual hosts, others can cause a range of respiratory or other symptoms. Sporadically, viruses spread across species, sometimes changing their genetics and surface molecules. Prevention involves vaccination against known strains; improving hygiene; humane farming; eliminating the use of live poultry markets; and culling infected animals in severe outbreaks.

infected by a bacteria later called *Salmonella*. And, in 1877, a new bird disease was identified called 'fowl plague', which would later be known as 'avian influenza' or 'bird flu' (Box 4).

Modern battlefields

At the start of the 20th century, many human societies and economies relied on horses, donkeys, and mules for agriculture and transportation—as several African, Asian, and Latin American communities still do today. This work often caused the animals a variety of injuries and health problems that not only made them

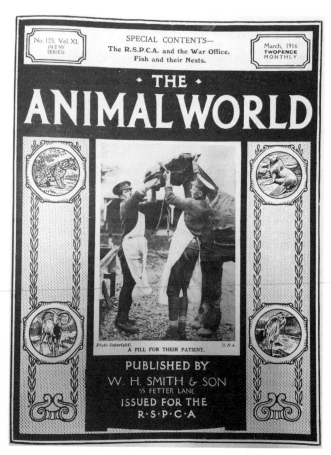

4. Cover of a contemporary magazine showing the treatment of a horse from the front in the First World War.

suffer but also reduced their economic usefulness. The First World War conscripted millions of horses for cavalry, artillery, and military transportation, who, like the men serving on the front, suffered from injuries, starvation, drowning, disease, and fatigue. Keeping them in active service became a central role for veterinarians, particularly on the Western Front where over two million horses were treated—and then returned to duty (Figure 4). Many armies even created their own dedicated veterinary army corps that continue today.

The health of farm animals also remained an important, if secondary, priority for veterinary scientists and practitioners. Veterinarians spent much of their time caring for individual cows, sheep, horses, and pigs. Those familiar with the stories of the famous English vet Alf Wight (best known by his *nom-de-plume* 'James Herriot') in his delightful *All Creatures Great and Small*, and its sequels, will appreciate the daily work of caring for individual animals. Veterinary science was seen as vital to supporting the performance of our farming industry, and to keeping humans safe from the animal produce they eat and drink. The Second World War took more plough-horses (and men) from farms and created food shortages. Recovering countries needed to increase their food production with limited horse and human labour.

In the subsequent peacetime, farmers began to increase the productivity of their land. They used by-products of the wars to increase their yield, such as tractors, pesticides based on chemical weapons, and nitrogen-based fertilizers chemically similar to explosives. These developments allowed farmers to produce more crops such as corn and soya that could be fed to farmed animals. Farmers (or, more accurately, breeding companies) created animals who grew faster or produced more eggs, milk, or offspring. Farms were re-designed to use more machines and fewer stockpersons. More animals were fitted into smaller spaces, for example putting hens in stacked cages or tying sows into stalls. And animals were prevented from wasting their calories through behavioural restrictions and social isolation.

These efforts had a big impact on how much each animal could provide. The daily milk yield of dairy cows has gone up considerably since the Second World War—arguably at the expense of their health (although, insofar as their lifespan is now limited, their total lifetime yields have not necessarily seen such rises). In that time, the growth of broiler chickens has sped up so much that they have reached slaughter weight one day earlier each year—they are now killed at well under 2 months old. And this process of increasing productivity has continued: in the last decade of the last century, numbers of poultry, pigs, and fish have vastly increased in many countries. Within the last few years, the volume of seafood produced in aquaculture systems exceeded wild caught stocks for the first time and, now, around 55 per cent of Atlantic salmon sold is from farmed rather than wild caught stocks.

The changes had mixed effects in terms of animal health. Keeping animals in smaller cages or stalls allowed farmers to control their environments more precisely. Keeping them indoors reduced their exposure to outdoor parasites. Putting animals on wire or slatted floors meant their faeces could drop straight into slurry pits, reducing the need for absorbent bedding that could harbour microbes. Keeping animals tied up or caged reduced the risks of injuries to themselves or one another. However, such farming also increased the risks of some infectious or mental health problems. So veterinary scientists looked for ways to prevent these problems while still keeping the animals in similar conditions. Some veterinary scientists developed vaccines to some common microbes (particularly viruses) such as Newcastle disease, a bird virus related to cattle plague that can cause respiratory and neurological problems in birds, particularly in chickens and pigeons, and occasionally in humans. Others found that giving antibiotics not only prevented some diseases, but could also make animals grow even faster.

The 20th century even saw the elimination of some diseases. The use of inoculations helped eradicate smallpox in humans. The Office International des Epizooties (OIE) was established to agree international trading rules regarding contagious livestock diseases like cattle plague. Later it would help coordinate the global eradication of cattle plague, alongside the United Nations' (UN's) Food and Agriculture Organization (FAO) and the Inter-African Bureau of Epizootic Diseases. In Kenya, the veterinary scientist Walter Plowright developed a cheap vaccine against cattle plague, based on techniques used for human polio vaccines. Through such efforts, cattle plague was eradicated worldwide—the last case was in Kenya in 2001. Many individual countries also managed to eradicate specific disease such as rabies, classical swine fever, and foot and mouth disease, although these still continue to cause problems elsewhere, and occasionally occur in officially disease-free countries such as the devastating outbreak in England in 2001.

Increasing attention was also given to the health risks that animal interactions posed to the humans. In 1945, James Steele, an American veterinary scientist, began a veterinary course in Washington that, once it moved to Atlanta, became the Center for Disease Control (CDC). Through the century, there were public scares about the contamination of meat by chemicals given to animals (e.g. steroids) and pollutants that can persist in the environment and be taken up by animals and, ultimately, humans (e.g. dioxine). Farmers and cows in Europe suffered from an outbreak of a fatal cattle disease related to scrapie in sheep and Creutzfeldt-Jakob disease in humans. This was bovine spongiform encephalopathy (BSE) or 'mad cow disease', so called because it could make cows nervous, trembly, mal-coordinated, reluctant to be milked, or even aggressive. In the UK, around 40,000 cows were killed in 1992 alone, devastating many farmers' lives, and severely damaging the British dairy and beef industries.

Veterinary science off the fields

The 20th century also saw an increasing veterinary attention given to animals other than the species used in farming and transportation. In 1908, the French scientists Charles Jules

Henry Nicolle (1866–1936) and Charles Comte (1869–1943) identified that *Leishmania* parasites could infect dogs (Box 5). Scientific work between the wars developed vaccines for dogs against distemper, particularly through work on both canine and human influenza, funded by dog owners. For much of the century, the veterinary care of pets continued to lack the status of large animal work: a 1938 UK report concluded that it 'could not justify expenditure of public money on the training of women for work among dogs and cats'. But, after the world wars, pet owners increasingly called on veterinary science to help their beloved pets: even James Herriot had to treat pets such as 'Tricky Woo', an over-fed lapdog to whom he had to speak like a human child. As the century progressed, companion animal veterinary work became the largest area of veterinary medicine in many countries.

Improved veterinary care perhaps allowed pet breeding to be relatively unfettered from concerns for the animals' health. Veterinary scientific studies suggest that probably all common dog breeds developed some unhealthy body shapes and genetic disorders. Ironically, treating these diseases helped to drive progress in veterinary science. This progress made veterinary science become increasingly aware of these diseases and their genetic causes. Concern over dog breeding eventually led to veterinary scientists and responsible breeders starting to try and reduce the health risks of controlled breeding. Between the wars and since, several health schemes have been introduced to reduce particular genetic problems, and efforts made to educate breeders, show

Box 5 Leishmaniasis

Leishmania microbes are spread by sandflies, particularly to dogs and humans. It is common in southern Europe, Africa, Asia, and South and Central America. It can cause skin lesions, eye problems, and organ failure. Treatment is variable and patients may continue to carry the microbes afterwards.

judges, and would-be pet owners to try to avoid such problems. To date, these have had disappointingly limited success.

The 20th century also saw major advances in our understanding of animals' biology, through studies of them both in the laboratory and in their environments. Hans Selye identified how animals often respond to a variety of different threats to their health, describing this general type of response as 'stress' that is reasonably consistent across a wide range of species, including reptiles and fish. Walter Bradford Cannon described ways in which animals' bodies can correct deviations from their bodies' normal function caused by external challenges, in order to sustain a relatively consistent balance, and described how animals respond to threats by 'fight or flight' in his book *Bodily Changes in Pain, Hunger, Fear and Rage: An Account of Recent Researches into the Function of Emotional Excitement*. This work was clearly inspired by concern for animals' experiences, albeit often described in behavioural terms.

Developing the prior work of scientists such as Ivan Pavlov, comparative psychologists such as J. B. Watson and B. F. Skinner studied how rats and human children interacted with their environment through their behaviour, while trying to ignore their feelings and experiences. Later scientists such as Konrad Lorenz, Nikolaas Tinbergen, and Karl von Frisch studied various behaviours shown by animals, exploring the complex reasons for that behaviour. Finally, in the second half of the century, scientists began to consider animals' feelings more explicitly—starting with humans and other apes, most famously in Jane Goodall's studies on chimpanzee communities.

Studies on animals' minds and behaviour complemented traditional veterinary science in developing a scientific approach to compassion. Inside and outside the laboratory, the last few decades of the 20th century saw the beginnings of an increased worldwide concern about animals' mental health and how they experience their environments. Animal welfare science showed that the methods by which modern farming keeps animals can have significant impacts on their mental health. It turned out that animals need to perform many of the behaviours prevented within some farms, laboratory cages, zoological collections, or animal shelters—and can suffer stress or poor physical or mental health when prevented from doing so.

Partly as a consequence of these concerns, the 20th century also saw major developments in veterinary care for laboratory animals. Laboratory animals could suffer diseases such as Sendai, another virus related to cattle plague. Scientists realized that ill animals often gave less reliable scientific results. So, after the Second World War, scientists began to breed laboratory animals by Caesarean section and keep them in sterile conditions to decrease infections. However, later in the century, scientists began to recognize that keeping animals in such stripped back conditions can lead to boredom and stress. Such mental health issues can also themselves lead to less accurate data. This may be one reason why data from animal tests have often been disappointingly poor at leading to new treatments for human (or animal) patients—who live very different lives to those laboratory animals.

Another major development of the 20th century was the environmental movement and concern for wild animal health. Birds caught in major oil spills needed to be rescued, cleaned, treated, and rehabilitated. Writers such as Aldo Leopold and David Ehrenfeld considered how humans might protect the health of ecosystems and our environments. Newly discovered chemicals such as polychlorinated biphenyl and DDT were found to accumulate in predators (as reported, for example, by Rachel Carson in her book *Silent Spring*), eventually leading to bans in many countries. Major disasters affected humans and other animals, such as 1984's Ethiopian famine and the Bhopal gas leak from a pesticide factory, which killed thousands of humans and animals. More positively, the century also saw several national and international efforts to limit global climate changes, albeit with varying degrees of optimism.

A late development of the last few decades of the 20th century was the start of the digital revolution. The veterinary profession, like its sister profession, has not always been particularly quick to embrace the opportunities provided by mainstream digital technologies. Nevertheless, mobile telecommunications and data-managing software have the potential to render decision-making more efficient, reduce human error, utilize 'big data' across farms, and fit in with owners' busy lives. The challenge is to capitalize on these advantages while ensuring they do not allow owners to treat their pets without veterinary expertise, or make treatments so expensive they can only be afforded by wealthy pet owners and large-scale commercial farming companies, disadvantaging subsistence farmers and developing countries. The opportunities are that these owners, and their animals, are the very ones whom telecommunication and digital advances can help most.

New and old diseases

The 20th century saw a number of new diseases come to the fore. Some were probably completely new, others re-emerged, others have only now been recognized for the first time. For example, between the world wars, a new disease related to classical swine fever was found in Kenya, spreading within Africa (hence its name, African swine fever), and then to Europe, Russia, Cuba, and the Caribbean. In the Great Rift Valley, Rift Valley fever was identified by workers in a veterinary laboratory in Kenya (Box 6). In Uganda, West Nile virus was found in a woman and Zika virus in a monkey (Box 7). In the Côte d'Ivoire, a new virus was found in goats and sheep, which was also related to cattle plague and caused symptoms so similar to the latter that it was called 'goat plague' or *peste des petits ruminants.*

Box 6 West Nile virus

This virus is transmitted by mosquitoes between animals including horses, crows, geese, alligators, and humans. It can cause neurological problems including mal-coordination and paralysis, and can be fatal. There are vaccines for birds, but a key prevention is restricting mosquito access where possible.

Box 7 Rift Valley fever

This virus can be spread across sheep, cows, buffalo, camels, and humans by mosquitoes, or by inhalation or contamination. In some species, it can cause miscarriages, liver or other problems, and death. Prevention involves vaccination, or by trying to predict and prevent outbreaks—for example, after flooding increases its spread by mosquitoes.

In the 1950s and 1960s, myxomatosis, which had been discovered in Uruguay in the 19th century, was deliberately spread to Australia and Europe in order to help control rabbit populations. Toxoplasmosis was identified as the cause of miscarriages in sheep (Box 8). In Japan, mercury from industrial water pollution caused neurological problems in cats, pigs, dogs, and humans. Measles (another disease related to cattle plague) was found to have infected laboratory rhesus monkeys in laboratories. As the decade ended, a new strain of avian influenza called H5 (due to one of its molecules) was discovered and a type of influenza virus was found to be a cause of respiratory problems in horses. In this decade, Ruth Harrison also first described some mental health conditions in animals farmed using the new methods in a book entitled *Animal Machines*, which helped to prompt the development of animal welfare science.

Box 8 Toxoplasmosis

Toxoplasma microbes mainly infect cats, but can also spread to other birds and mammals. They are spread by eating uncooked meat, infected faeces, or through the placenta. Toxoplasmosis often causes no problems, but can sometimes be fatal. In humans, the key concerns are miscarriage, retinal problems, and death. Prevention links to worming cats, avoiding cat faeces, washing our hands, and cooking meat.

Box 9 Borreliosis (Lyme disease)

Different species of *Borrelia* bacteria are spread by ticks in and between many host species, including dogs, humans, and birds (and many other species that may carry the ticks), causing various symptoms. Borreliosis can be treated using antibiotics but may leave patients with ongoing infections.

In the 1970s, lumpy skin disease—a pox virus that causes (unsurprisingly) lumpy skin in cattle—spread from buffalo in southern and eastern Africa into sub-Saharan west Africa. Humans suffered from a new and confusing disease in Lyme, Connecticut (Box 9). In 1974, koi sleepy disease was first reported in fish in Japan and pig circovirus was discovered (although it was not until the 1990s that a new type would cause widespread problems of wasting, and reproductive, and probably kidney and skin, disease). In the late 1970s, dogs began to get severe diarrhoea from a new canine parvovirus that probably came from cats (who can also get a parvoviral diarrhoea) and, in Korea, hantavirus was identified as infecting rats and humans, potentially causing pain, fever, bleeding, and kidney problems.

The 1970s also saw the emergence of a virus in red squirrels in England, that was found, in the early 1980s, to be a pox virus related to the Variola virus that causes smallpox in humans. A new virus was found in pigs that caused a reproductive and respiratory syndrome (called porcine reproductive and respiratory syndrome (PRRS)). A strain of *Salmonella* emerged and spread worldwide, becoming resistant to various drugs. In the late 1980s, thousands of seals died from a new virus related to cattle plague, and thousands more died from the distemper virus found in dogs.

In the 1990s, alongside the emergence of BSE, various new viruses were identified such as koi herpes. Several 'new' viruses related to cattle plague were discovered in porpoises, dolphins, and whales; in humans and horses (found in 1994 in Hendra, Australia); and in humans and pigs (in Nipah, Malaysia in 1998) (Box 10). The latter outbreak killed around a hundred humans, and over a million pigs were culled in efforts to control the disease. In 1998, Chytridiomycosis, a disease caused by the fungus *Batrachochytrium dendrobatidis*, was found in amphibians as it spread worldwide. The late 1990s and early 2000s also saw various strains of avian influenza, some of them especially dangerous, which particularly spread in Southeast Asia through live animal markets.

Also in the 2000s, sudden acute respiratory syndrome (SARS) was identified in China among animal and meat traders associated

Box 10 Hendra and Nipah

These related viruses can infect pigs (Hendra), horses (Nipah), humans, and bats. They can cause neurological or respiratory problems and up to 75 per cent mortality depending on species, with no known cure. There is now a vaccine for Hendra, but the key prevention methods include reducing their spread by humane farming, understanding and avoiding optimum disease-inducing ecology, avoiding disrupting bat colonies, and the use of protective equipment.

with a live animal market that sold masked palm civets, raccoon dogs, and Chinese ferret badgers. In the USA, an outbreak of monkeypox occurred in 2003, brought into the country with some Gambian pouched rats and prairie dogs sold as exotic pets. In 2006, a white fungal disease was found growing on the muzzles and wings of North American bats, later termed 'white nose syndrome', that has now killed millions of bats. In 2009, a strain of influenza emerged that was a combination of three types—human, pig, and bird.

In the last few years, Middle East respiratory syndrome (MERS) has been identified in Saudi Arabia. This is a similar disease to SARS, perhaps having come to humans from one-humped camels. New viruses related to cattle plague have also been found in cats and vampire bats. In 2014, there was a major outbreak of Ebola. One suggestion has been that the first human patient became infected while playing in a hollow tree that housed a colony of Angolan free-tailed bats and there is continued suspicion that humans have been infected by eating bushmeat. And from 2013, Zika virus was reported as causing widespread human embryo problems in the Pacific Islands and then Brazil. There was also a resurgence of leprosy in UK red squirrels.

Fortunately, some of these diseases are being slowly eradicated. Inspired by the eradication of cattle plague, the FAO of the UN and the OIE have just produced a global strategy to control and eradicate goat plague by 2030 (helped, perhaps less predictably, by the International Atomic Energy Agency). Brucellosis, which causes spontaneous abortion in cattle, and foot and mouth disease have been largely eliminated from many countries. Human tuberculosis from cows' milk is largely eliminated in many countries through pasteurization (other human cases come from different bacteria spread by humans, or very rarely by voles). Rabies has been slowly eradicated across Europe and areas of North America, and was never present in Australia. Recently, the OIE has established banks of dog vaccines to use alongside vaccines given to wild carnivores in food with the ambition of eradicating rabies by 2030.

However, many of these diseases continue to have an impact today. The World Health Organization (WHO) still reported 783 human cases of bubonic 'plague' in 2013, alongside untold numbers of rodent deaths. While smallpox is eradicated, cowpox is still found in rodents, cats who catch the rodents, and owners who pet the cats; and monkeypox is found in humans and other primates in Africa, and sometimes elsewhere after the international movement of infected exotic pets. *Leishmania* continues to infect thousands of dogs and humans across all major continents, particularly in under-nourished children or HIV infected people. Rabies kills tens of thousands of people each year, plus uncounted dogs and other animals.

Tuberculosis—from cows and humans—continues to infect animals and humans in some developing countries. Goat plague has rapidly spread through Africa and across the Middle East and Asia—to China in 2007, Morocco in 2008, Georgia in February, and the Maldives in April 2016. Goat plague causes losses of around US$1.5 billion annually, particularly in developing African and South Asian countries. West Nile virus has spread around Africa, Asia, Europe, North America, and, more recently, into Australia, Latin America, South America, and the Caribbean. Lumpy skin disease has spread through the Middle East to Turkey, Greece, Macedonia, and, in April 2016, to Bulgaria. PRRS has spread worldwide and, in Asia and the USA, the virus appears to have mutated, making it harder to control. Foot and mouth disease and swine fever still occur in many countries, as do other diseases such as brucellosis and Rift Valley fever. And a new case of BSE was reported as recently as 2015 in Canada.

Veterinary science today

Nowadays, veterinary science is both scientific and clinical. As a scientific field, it encompasses the biology—physiology, pathology, behaviour, and psychology—of over a million species of animals. As a clinical subject, veterinary science covers the treatment—diagnostics, medicine, surgery, and care—of billions of animals. It is a vital support to modern farming, animal research, pet-keeping, and conservation, helping millions of owners and consumers. (Occasionally, slightly provocative veterinary scientists like to contrast this with the single species and thirty-two teeth covered by their sister professionals in human medical and dental sciences.)

Most veterinary patients (as with their owners and consumers) are vertebrates, particularly mammals, birds, reptiles, and bony fish, but veterinarians may also often be faced with invertebrates such as bees and corals. Other invertebrates, such as tapeworms and lice, are more usually considered medical enemies rather than patients, and veterinary science studies these animals mainly to understand how to then treat their victims. Only one animal species is outside veterinary science—*Homo sapiens*—although there are many important cross-overs between humans and other animals. In this book, the term 'animal', and the pronoun 'we', will be used to include human and non-human members of the same kingdom.

At its very core, veterinary science is about animal health or, in other words, animals' physical, mental, and social well-being. Physical well-being comes from having the ability to grow and sustain one's body, and to avoid major disabilities, injuries, and infections. Mental well-being comes from having the ability to process environmental stimuli and emotions appropriately, and to avoid states such as stress, depression, and prolonged anxiety. Social well-being comes from having the right company, and the ability to avoid such feelings as fear, isolation, and loneliness. Health is also a positive concept—good physical, mental, and social well-being will be attained when animals can fulfil their motivations and enjoy their environments. Veterinary science not only aims to minimize suffering but also to ensure animals get enough opportunities for good quality, fulfilled lives, unfrustrated by disabilities or impoverished resources.

Veterinary science is ultimately about what is good for the animals—not just what is good for humans in terms of meat, eggs, data, or companionship (although these may also be important). Other scientists may alter or use animals purely for human benefits, for example to develop human medicines or increase farm productivity. Such efforts may or may not be laudable in each case—but they are arguably not 'veterinary' any more than equivalent uses of human subjects would be considered 'medical'. As an illustration, making animals ill for laboratory studies on human diseases is *not* veterinary science—but subsequently studying how to make those animals well again arguably *is*.

Within this focus, veterinary science also serves a much wider range of human aims. It can help improve human health by reducing the spread of diseases across species, improving the nutritional value of animal produce, and developing medicines that can be applied to human patients. It can help human economics by increasing the productivity of farming, improving land use, and reducing poverty. It can enhance social justice by improving food security and sustaining subsistence farmers and herdsmen. And it can help protect the environment by reducing pollution and greenhouse emissions, and supporting wild populations. Having healthy animals in good environments can help achieve these aims and make animal lives better too. These multiple aims—with animal welfare as a priority—are reflected in the oaths that many veterinarians in many countries are now asked to swear (Box 11).

Because of its wide scope, many contributions to veterinary science have come from researchers who are not qualified veterinarians—including biologists, chemists, nutritionists, behaviourists, psychologists, ecologists, and farriers. Furthermore, many applications of veterinary care are provided by non-veterinarians. Veterinary nurses and technicians play an

Box 11 A common veterinary oath

Being admitted to the profession of veterinary medicine,
I solemnly swear to use my scientific knowledge and skills for
the benefit of society through the protection of animal health
and welfare, the prevention and relief of animal suffering, the
conservation of animal resources, the promotion of public
health, and the advancement of medical knowledge. I will
practise my profession conscientiously, with dignity, and in
keeping with the principles of veterinary medical ethics. I accept
as a lifelong obligation the continual improvement of my
professional knowledge and competence.

increasingly important and professional role. Owners and
stockpersons have to notice signs of illness, sometimes administer
treatment (hopefully under veterinary advice), and, most
importantly, prevent disease by providing the animals in their
charge with a good diet and environment. This book takes an
inclusive scope of 'veterinary science' in order to help us
understand the shared values, scientific overlaps, and myriad
interconnections across species and disciplines.

Increasingly, veterinary science is overlapping with other fields—
in particular with biomedical, food, and ecological sciences. Many
scientific efforts contribute to veterinary science as well as other
fields of scientific discovery, while veterinary science can inform
other fields too. Doctors trying to protect human health need to
understand animal nutrition and the transfer of disease between
species, helping to translate advanced practices from human to
animal patients. Food scientists trying to maintain food quality
and security need to take account of the health, stress, genetics,
and production system of the animals humans eat, while ensuring
the animals themselves have the right care and nutrition.

Ecologists need to evaluate the impact of farming methods and animal diseases on the global environment, and help determine the effects of animal movements and environmental changes. There is a lot at stake—for humans and animals—in reaching the right level of coordination across disciplines, meaning that experts need to fully understand one another's fields.

Chapter 2
Our families and other animals

Animal medicine

Most of us are familiar with medicine for human patients. Some of us may be registered doctors who treat human patients. Most of us are human patients. Many of us even provide some medicine for ourselves and our human families, self-diagnosing medical conditions and even administering treatments such as aspirin. News articles present promising 'breakthroughs' in medical science, which are often based on data from animal research. And our lives and decisions can be coloured by concern for our families' health, and the threat of future illness, pain, and death. Maintaining our own health is so central to our lives that it is called 'medicine'—when, to be more specific, it might be better called something like 'anthropic medicine'.

In comparison, most of us are generally less *au fait* with veterinary medicine. This is perhaps surprising. Some of us are farmers or breeders, or work in pet-shops, zoos, circuses, or laboratories. Many of us look after pets. Most of us eat animals or their products, and use drugs developed in animal research. All of us live close to a variety of urban or rural wildlife, and in local environments and a global climate that are affected by, and affect, the animals who live in them. So all our lives depend on veterinary medical science to keep us safe, nourished, and happy. But we are often oblivious to how veterinary science is providing for our needs and keeping us humans healthy.

An understanding of anthropic medical science can help us understand veterinary medical science. Veterinary science and healthcare relate to non-human animal patients in similar ways to how anthropic science and healthcare relate to human patients. Those involved in each field investigate similar diseases and biological processes. They diagnose and treat similar conditions in their patients, and give similar advice to clients. Anthropic and veterinary medical science overlap considerably, and can learn from one another. There are important differences that clinicians must take into account, although many of these might be considered cultural, linguistic, or even socio-political differences.

But it is not that helpful simply to compare and contrast anthropic and veterinary science. The fields can be better considered as two sides of a coin, or two parallel lenses to explore a single, over-arching scientific field. Anthropic and veterinary scientists working together has the promise of significant potential benefits—for human and non-human patients—so long as everyone involved can genuinely understand, and care about, the aims and theories within the fields. 'Medical science'—and related concepts like 'patient' and, in many countries, 'doctor'—applies to all animals. To put it simply: veterinary science is *part* of medical science.

This is because, fundamentally, humans *are* animals. We—meaning all animals—share similarities in our fundamental biology, the diseases we can get, our responses to those diseases, and our responses to treatments. Understanding *animal* biology means understanding humans and other animals. Indeed, it is our similarities that explain why scientists use non-human animals to develop treatments, why companies want to test whether drugs and other chemicals are effective and safe in other species before humans use them, and why veterinary scientists adapt cutting-edge anthropic treatments. Indeed, there is a cycle in anthropic and veterinary medical science. Many drugs are initially given to non-human animal subjects experimentally, then (if promising) given to human patients, then adapted for non-human animal patients. The exact species may differ: the laboratory animals are usually rodents and fish, while the animal patients are often dogs, cats, and horses—as most owners do not spend so much on their mice, rats, or zebrafish. There is a complex scientific interconnection and mutual dependency across species.

In fact, veterinary science itself is, in its very essence, a cross-species science. The wide range of patients helps veterinary scientists to understand medical biology on a fundamental level, recognizing meaningful similarities between species and understanding significant differences. They can apply general biological concepts and techniques to all species, such as basic principles of disease control and surgical hygiene. They can adapt their learning from diseases seen in familiar animals to generate working hypotheses about unstudied illnesses in rarer animals. Treatments for domestic cows or dogs might be cautiously trialled in the hope they will help aurochs or raccoon dogs. This also allows veterinary scientists to have particular insights into human biology, essentially because humans are one (more) animal species of many that veterinarians treat.

Understanding medical biology on a fundamental level also helps to recognize what are relevant differences across species. Veterinary medicine, in its very essence, is also a comparative science. Different species may have a variety of body shapes, biological processes, behaviour, and diseases. Guinea pigs' and hamsters' beneficial (or 'friendly') gut bacteria can be killed off by penicillin, allowing harmful microbes to multiply and make them even more ill. Raccoon dogs may suffer mental health issues in domestic homes that dogs do not. What is medicine for the goose is not necessarily medicine for the gander. Alongside 'human–animal differences', there are greater differences between

33

horses and seahorses than between horses and humans (let alone closely related apes). There are also many differences within species, between bloodlines, genders, patients, and each individual over time.

Animal biology: anatomy, physiology, and genetics

A good starting point for veterinary science is the study of animals' bodies. As Chapter 1 described, anatomists have long studied the structure of animals' bodies: from the overall construction of our skeletons and major organs, through the composition of the tissues that make up those organs, and the makeup of individual cells, even down to micro-anatomy of the structures within those cells. Meanwhile physiologists and biochemists have studied how our bodies function, from the electrical pathways of our nerves to the chemical pathways in our cells. Geneticists have identified the coding that directs what proteins are produced in our cells, which then affect our anatomy, physiology, and behaviour.

All living vertebrates—mammals, birds, reptiles, amphibians, and fish—have common ancestors, who lived around 500–600 million years ago. All vertebrates share many (around 10,000) genes that code for common features: multi-chambered hearts; teeth; internal bones and cartilage; and specialized hormonal and immune systems, including pancreas, thymus, adrenal, pituitary, and thyroid glands. This means all vertebrates share similar basic biological needs to grow, develop, and sustain our bodies healthily. As Boyle and Hooke horridly showed, every animal requires oxygen. They also need an adequate diet with enough protein, fat, carbohydrates, minerals, and vitamins; and enough space and resources to exercise their motivated behaviours. Each animal needs adequate shelter from the heat and cold, safe water and decent air quality, and the ability to avoid threat from other animals, poisons, and injuries. Mammals, birds, reptiles, amphibians, and fish all need fundamentally similar conditions to live and to thrive.

Of course, it does not need a veterinary scientist to see that the specifics may vary between species. Veterinary patients may have none, one, two, four, six, or eight legs. They may have beaks, hooves, or claws; and fur, feathers, or scales. They may give birth to live young or lay eggs. They may walk, swim, burrow, or fly. They may live on land or in the water. They may live in complex groups or nearly always alone. Some have quite short lifespans such as Syrian hamsters who usually only live a year or so and brown antichinuses who die after their first two-week breeding season. Others can live for many decades, such as Galápagos tortoises who can reportedly live to 170 years. Some survive the desert heat, such as fennec foxes. Others can survive below freezing, such as amphibians and fish who seem to produce a natural antifreeze (although ice crystals in their bodies may cause other health problems).

This means that animals' precise needs may differ. Diet is a good example. Green tree frogs eat only meat (except any vegetation in their prey's intestines). Goats eat only plants (except any unlucky invertebrate eaten accidentally). Rabbits and horses have teeth that need enough chewing to wear them down as they constantly grow. Cows, goats, and sheep have large stomachs containing ecosystems of hundreds of different microbes, which themselves have specific nutritional needs. Many species of snake can usually obtain enough vitamin D from their meat-based diet, while many lizards can synthesize it in their skin under sunlight or manmade UV lights. Most animals can also synthesize vitamin C, except humans and guinea pigs who need it ready-made from their diet.

Our species (and, more generally, our genes) are important determinants of our biology. But—fortunately for my daughter—our bodies are not completely determined by our genes. They often depend on how our genes interact with our environments. It is the interactions between genes and the environment—and, more generally, between animals and their environments—that determines each animal's biology. Our genes, bodies, behaviour, and environments affect one another in complex ways. For example, a lack of food can affect how our genes are expressed (i.e. what effect they have on our hormones and our behaviour). Animals need to 'fit' our environments to survive and even more so to thrive in them. *Mens sana in corpore sano—in tuto sancto*.

Animal diseases: pathology and microbiology

Our biological similarities mean that animals may get a range of broadly similar diseases. Glands may produce too little or too much of a hormone. Brains may spontaneously misfire in epileptic seizures. Joints, brains, and kidneys may degenerate over time. Cells may grow abnormally, causing tumours or cancers. Short noses can make breathing difficult.

Many of these malfunctions may be coded into animals' genes. For example, humans and cats can both have variations such as Klinefelter syndrome whereby their cells contain two 'X' and one 'Y' chromosomes, which often causes no problems but can lead to developmental abnormalities or infertility. Veterinary scientists have also identified cat genes associated with heart-muscle thickening and kidney cysts. Breeding chickens or turkeys for fast growth in commercial farms can be linked to weaker immune responses, lameness, dropsy, Newcastle disease, and sudden death. Some bloodlines of Dalmatians are at particular risk of deafness or bladder stones. Others seem to have high risks of various cancers, such as Boxers, Golden Retrievers, and Rottweilers. Many dog, cat, and sheep breeds have squashed noses.

Many diseases involve infections and infestations of microbes or parasites. Some live on animals' bodies, including arachnids like fleas and mites, bacteria like *Staphylococcus aureus*, and fungi such as ringworm. Others live inside animals, including worms like tapeworms and flukes, single-celled protozoa like Trypanosomes and other bacteria such as *E. coli* and *Salmonella*.

Some reproduce inside cells, including bacteria like *Chlamydia* and viruses like influenza and parvoviruses. Other diseases such as BSE and scrapie are caused by misshapen proteins that somehow disrupt other proteins, somewhat like Kurt Vonnegut's fictional *ice-nine* substance that causes water to freeze at room temperature and build up in brain tissue. Some microbes and parasites are quite generalist, such as some *Salmonella* strains. Others are more specialist, such as the flukes *Diplostomum spathacaeum* and *Cymothoa exigua* that are precisely adapted to develop in fish eyes or in place of a fish's tongue.

However, microbes aren't all bad all the time. Some live on, in, or around us harmlessly, and only make us ill when something goes wrong. For example, the bacteria that cause botulism or tetanus can live harmlessly in the environment, in animal intestines, or on our skin—it is when they get under our skin (usually through a wound), or we eat them, that the toxic chemicals they produce lead to neurological issues such as lockjaw or weakness. Similarly, the fungus that causes white nose syndrome in bats may be able to survive on cave walls, living on decaying matter, but can cause highly fatal outbreaks.

Some microbes are even beneficial. All animals have large numbers of microbes that live on our skin, in our guts, and in our respiratory tracts. They help our digestion: indeed, cows cannot survive if the microbes that digest grass in their intestines are killed off by antibiotics. They help defend us from other microbes that could cause us disease: bacteria in humans' noses were recently found to produce a potential new type of antibiotic. They can help keep our environments safe and clean (e.g. the bacteria that use up fish waste products to maintain water quality). Nevertheless, some of these bacteria may still sometimes cause problems, if their host is otherwise ill or they build up to overly large numbers.

Other health problems are not caused by microbes, but by how animals live. An excessive intake of calories and insufficient exercise can cause obesity in most species—which is now common among pet and show animals, for example affecting potentially between 22 per cent and 40 per cent of pet dogs worldwide. Car accidents or physical violence can cause broken bones and internal bleeding. High temperatures can cause burns or hyperthermia. Chemicals can cause poisoning or reactions. Sometimes what causes disease in one animal may be unproblematic for another and it is often the combination of the genes and the environment that leads to illness. For example, humans can tolerate chemicals in chocolate, ibuprofen, and grapes that can be highly toxic to dogs.

Of course, different animals do not all get the same diseases. Humans seem particularly prone to atherosclerosis, prostate disease, and dental caries (as are other captive apes). Horses are very susceptible to tetanus, compared to pigs, dogs, and cats. Rats are prone to some mammary tumours. Many farm animals are slaughtered before they are old enough to suffer some of the diseases relating to old age, whereas cancer is probably the main medical cause of canine death in the USA, particularly in breeds with a genetic predisposition. Indeed, many purebred dog breeds each have a list of diseases to which they are prone. Similarly, some sheep breeds, and those with particular genes, seem to be at higher risk of certain forms of scrapie in the USA. Unlike adult humans, most domestic animals do not really get to choose their diet, lifestyle, partners, interactions, or environment, so their diseases are largely, or entirely, our fault.

Animal minds: psychology and ethology

Most vertebrate animals have basically similar nervous systems: long spinal cords to transmit signals through our bodies and well-developed brains with similar areas that appear to process our thoughts and feelings. Indeed, it is the older, shared parts of the brain that control basic processes and emotions that are particularly relevant to animals' mental health, behaviour, and well-being. Reptiles, fish, birds, and mammals all have brain areas that function very similarly to those areas in humans that correspond to our experiences. Humans, dolphins, and whales have larger brains overall, but there is no good reason to consider other animals less able to suffer when they are ill. In fact, since they have fewer psychological coping mechanisms, they might actually suffer more in some situations.

Most animals seem to experience unpleasant feelings such as pain, itchiness, nausea, malaise, confusion, distress, restlessness, loneliness, boredom, irritability, anxiety, and fear. These may be linked to illnesses or to particular sources of stress such as impoverished environments. Furthermore, animal patients can also experience negative feelings associated with medical treatment itself, such as pain after surgery (including possible phantom limb pain), nausea from chemotherapy, or fear when visiting the hospital. Humans can also suffer from diseases that involve pain with no or few physical signs, such as headaches and fibromyalgia, or post-surgical conditions such as phantom limb pain—and it is very difficult to know when other animals might suffer from similar conditions.

A key way to study animals' emotions and mental processes is by observing behaviours that seem to be associated with emotional situations. Emotions might make animals behave aggressively, traumatize themselves, sleep badly, or avoid scary places (such as hospitals). Emotions may be linked to various visual (e.g. colour or postural changes), auditory (e.g. whining), or chemical (e.g. scents) signs. Humans, horses, cats, rodents, and other animals seem to show particular facial expressions when threatened, in pain, or stressed. Dogs may lower their tails when scared—although, contrary to popular belief, wagging tails probably suggests confusion or anxiety rather than happiness; or it could be that dogs learn to wag their tails because it prompts good reactions from human owners (although recent evidence suggests *how* dogs wag their tails may subtly show whether they see something they like or dislike).

However, most animals are not very good at recognizing the emotions of other species, perhaps particularly non-social species, for whom showing signs of illness has no benefit. Other animals may not show signs that other species can readily recognize. Prey species (i.e. most farm animals, pets and laboratory animals) may inhibit behavioural responses when there is a potential predator nearby. Since they may perceive humans as potential predators, this can mean owners and veterinarians struggle to identify signs of their illness. Veterinary scientists need to have enough humility to recognize our limitations, particularly for species less similar to ourselves such as fish, amphibians, and reptiles. Rather than illogically concluding that, because of human limitations in recognizing those emotions, they must not exist, veterinary scientists increasingly give animals the benefit of the doubt.

Our animal brains also put us at risk of neurological and mental health problems. Brain malfunctions can cause changes such as forgetfulness, seizures, or personality changes. These can cause unpleasant feelings such as confusion, disorientation, and behaviours such as toileting in the house, vocalizing abnormally, aggression, or repetitive behaviours. Of particular importance are stress, anxiety, and depression. Such conditions are not only unpleasant, but can also lead to other diseases. For example, stress can be linked to a weakened immune system, making the animals susceptible to infectious diseases. This is one reason why cows and horses may suddenly come down with respiratory diseases when they are transported for long distances.

Another mental health problem is when animals learn not to bother reacting to stresses—a condition known as 'learned apathy' or 'learned helplessness'. This was observed in rather unpleasant experiments in which dogs who were repeatedly given inescapable electric shocks learnt not to bother trying to avoid them. This apathy has been linked (in humans) to situations such as poor parenting, domestic violence, and poverty; (in farm and laboratory animals) to restrictive situations such as pigs in small stalls or crates; and perhaps (in horses) to painful or uncomfortable training methods. It may also be linked to depression.

Mental health problems might start because of genuine danger, frustration, or conflict, but then develop into more general anxiety syndromes, phobias, or compulsive/obsessive disorders. Others may begin with normal activities such as grooming, walking, digging, and hunting that become increasingly exaggerated or altered. Sometimes these issues are linked to our hormones, in particular to the hormones involved in stress. Long-term stress, tumours, or malfunctions of the glands can cause an over-production of stress hormones, which can lead to increased eating and toileting, panting, poor sleep, and anxiety. Some mental health problems may also have a (partly) genetic basis, sometimes predisposing individual animals to developing problems when their environments are imperfect.

Mental health conditions are sometimes considered primarily as 'behavioural' problems. Ethologists study animals' behaviour in order to understand those animals, and veterinary scientists often use behaviour to help diagnose illnesses. Sometimes certain behaviours are harmful in themselves (e.g. self-mutilation in monkeys or aggression in dogs), and often they are unwelcome for the owner (e.g. urinating in the house or barking—although some of these may be normal behaviours rather than signs of illness). Nevertheless, veterinary scientists need to consider these issues from the perspective of the patient—whose mental experience consists of the underlying emotions, not the behaviour. The study (and manipulation) of animal behaviour can be valuable, but the study or manipulation of the underlying mental states even more so.

Animal responses to diseases: immunology and pathophysiology

When animals sustain an injury or an illness, our bodies fight back. We detoxify poisons and excrete them in our urine or faeces.

We respond to stresses by changing our metabolism to be ready for action. We respond to infections by increasing our body temperature to inhibit bacterial growth: mammals and birds, by generating heat internally; and reptiles and fish, by moving to warmer areas. We make white blood cells and antibody proteins that can detect and attack chemicals on the surfaces of microbes, parasites, or cancer cells. We respond to injuries by making the tissues inflamed to help our defensive cells get to the microbes and damaged tissues.

Our immune responses are constantly getting rid of many microbes and cancerous cells well before they cause disease. Often they see them off completely. At other times, they may win only a partial victory, leaving some microbes or cells in the body that can cause chronic illness; or which lie low for a time and then flare back up. How well our bodies respond can alter what effect a disease has. Some diseases, such as leishmaniasis, can look very different depending on the success of the animal's immune response: patients may show no symptoms; may get ill but fully recover; have chronic skin, eye, or blood problems; develop kidney failure, vomiting, diarrhoea, or joint pain; or simply die. Our immune responses can depend on many factors, including our age, breed, genetics, nutrition, previous exposure, and other concurrent diseases.

We also respond to prevent further damage or pain. We may limp or become more sensitive, thus reducing any further damage to injured body parts. We may become sleepy, thus saving energy and keeping us out of sight of predators we would be too weak to escape. We may in the future learn to avoid foods or situations—or people—that made us ill or injured, thus avoiding repetitions. These changes are adaptive responses by the body, orchestrated by our immune, hormone, and nervous systems. They can change our very motivations so that we actually no longer want to eat, play, groom, or reproduce. Unfortunately, they often do so by making us feel rotten.

Our responses may also limit the spread of infection to others. One recent theory suggests that many of our behaviours when we are ill not only help us to fight the infection, but also stop us spreading the microbes further. Badgers and bats may leave their sett or roosting site when ill (and many pet owners report that their pets 'go off to die'), perhaps saving the rest of their group from infection. Rats appear able to smell certain infections in others, and thereby avoid them. Many species of animals may drink less, thereby reducing the contamination of water sources. Of course, some behaviours may have both effects: lethargy may both save energy and reduce the spread of disease.

Our bodily attempts to tackle diseases can also cause problems in themselves. Scratching, biting, or licking ourselves may make us ever more sore or itchy (Figure 5). The body may treat some of its own cells or chemicals as dangerous and try to get rid of them, causing autoimmune diseases. The cells involved in our immune responses may grow too fast or abnormally, causing cancers such as lymphomas. The immune system may 'over-react' to chemicals or cells that the body detects, causing allergies to foods, plants, dust, or hay moulds. Indeed, sometimes severe infections—which would be bad enough anyway—can trigger a widespread immune over-reaction, leading to a fever, low blood pressure, clots within blood vessels, internal bleeding, multiple organ failure, and, potentially, to anaphylactic or septic shock and death.

Our psychological responses might also become over-reactions. It is normal and appropriate for animals to fear genuine threats in a proportionate manner. But some animals might develop a phobia to situations that they connect to harmful events such as firework displays. Some dogs become scared of a person, or a type of person, after they have been abused. Many animals can develop general excessive or prolonged anxiety syndromes, where they are overly concerned with potential dangers. Animals faced with continued stress may perform behaviours to cope with the stress for so long that the behaviours become repetitive and ingrained.

43

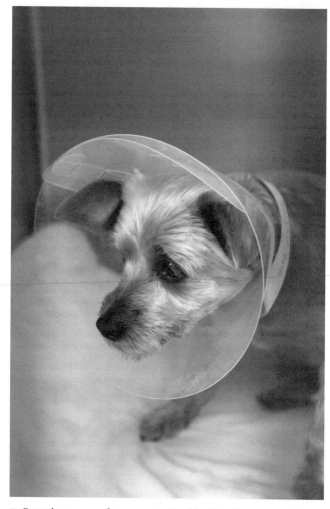

5. Sometimes we need to prevent animals' self-medicating responses, such as stopping them licking their wounds.

Arguably some of these reactions are appropriate responses
to horrible situations, but they are usually still unpleasant and
better avoided.

Chronic stress—due to repeated illness, injury, pain, or poor
environments—may, over time or during key developmental
phases, lead to changes in our hormonal and neurological processes.
Such stress can change the ways in which our bodies and brains
make the hormones and chemicals involved in our responses, such
as cortisol, dopamine, adrenaline, and serotonin. These changes
can alter the way in which we think and feel. Animals may become
generally stressed, anxious, or depressed. Indeed, there is evidence
that long-term physical problems, such as inflammation, can
damage animals' mental health. Conversely, severe or continued
stress can cause or exacerbate some physical diseases such as
cystitis, dermatitis, and intestinal problems. Animals' responses
to health problems can often be beneficial, but they have their
own consequences.

Diseases fight back

Animals' responses are not perfect—if they were then we would
never get ill. Animals may have poor responses to challenges when
they already have other health problems such as infections, some
tumours, severe burns, hypothermia, or malnutrition. Animals
may be unable to cope with stress, if their environment lacks
the resources they need, creating conflict or frustration, so
that they perform a similar behaviour towards an alternative
resource (e.g. pecking at other chickens when they cannot
forage); do something seemingly unrelated (e.g. urinating in
situations of stress) instead; or give up completely. Stress and
other health problems can also suppress animals' immune
responses to infections.

In fact, there are many reasons why some animals might not
mount successful immune responses. Young animals may not have

developed the capacity to produce their own antibodies to tackle the microbes they meet. Instead, they need to get the right antibodies from their mother via the egg contents or their first drinks of milk. When they do not get those antibodies, for example if they are separated from their mothers just after birth, they can be at risk of intestinal, respiratory, and other illnesses, if they are not managed correctly. Some medical conditions also limit animals' immune responses. Some pedigree cows, dogs, and cats are born without a functional thymus. Some humans, cats, mink, and killer whales have white blood cells that do not fight microbes properly. Some medications (e.g. steroids or cancer drugs) can also suppress animals' immune responses.

Sometimes our bodies simply do not recognize infections as being worth fighting. Our immune systems need to differentiate safe cells from dangerous infections: otherwise we would be constantly fighting our own cells, beneficial microbes, and food. However, this gives microbes and cancer cells a chance to avoid being noticed by our immune responses: for example some viruses may delay or pause their reproduction so as not to stimulate the immune response. This allows some infections or cancerous cells to remain latent, without any clinical signs of disease, sometimes for many years, until they finally cause full blown disease or spread to other animals. As we shall see, this can be a problem in determining how long to quarantine animals.

Over time, our immune systems can get better at recognizing and fighting particular microbes each time they encounter them—a process we may describe as 'becoming immune' to a disease. An individual's first, naive response to a microbe they have not encountered before may take a while to get going. But after we have encountered a microbe, our immune systems improve their ability to recognize them quickly. Specifically, our immune systems get better at recognizing particular molecules on the microbes, for example those to which antibodies attach. This readiness means we do not need to maintain large numbers of antibodies or to keep all our immune cells mobilized all the time, which would use up bodily resources and could itself cause disease from the effects of all those antibodies on our bodies. Instead, our bodies retain a smaller number in reserve that are ready to gear up, multiply, and attack when a familiar microbe enters the body.

However, microbes have ways to slow this improvement. Some microbes come in a wide variety, with different molecules on each, so we become immune to one type but remain vulnerable to others. Other microbes change what chemicals they present, so our immune systems no longer recognize them. There are over 2,500 different types of *Salmonella*, so we are unlikely to become immune to all of them, plus some types possess genes for many different surface molecules and can make different ones during different infections. Similar changes by Trypanosome parasites mean patients make repeated immune responses to multiple infections, which can build up toxic by-products that eventually make the patient comatose (hence the name of 'sleeping sickness' for one disease in humans). Influenza viruses can even mutate their genes, slightly changing the molecules on their surface, and generating virulent new strains of human, bird, and swine flu.

Other microbes stop the immune system attacking them. The rabies virus can hide within nervous tissues while it moves towards the brain (at up to 1cm per day). Mycobacteria and *Toxoplasma* parasites may get engulfed by white blood cells, but can then stop the cells from killing and digesting them. Bubonic plague bacteria appear able to reduce the immune responses of their victims, and can survive in some white blood cells and lymph nodes. Other microbes use various methods to weaken our immune systems, such as measles, distemper, African Swine Fever, PRRS, the group of immunodeficiency viruses found in cows, cats, pumas, monkeys, and humans, and related diseases in horses, sheep, and goats. As a result, animals with such conditions may die from a secondary infection with which their depleted immune system is unable to cope.

Some diseases can also alter our responses to them in order to increase the spread of infection. The microscopic parasite *Toxoplasma* and the fluke *Euhaplorchis californiensis* can cause infected rodents and killifish to behave differently so they are more likely to be eaten by cats and birds, respectively, who then get infected. The rabies virus can make some animals more aggressive—the classic 'rabid dog'—so that they bite other animals and thereby spread the disease. Bubonic plague bacteria may weaken fleas so that they are more likely to push bacteria into animals instead of sucking blood out. Mice can get a virus that makes infected cells reproduce rapidly, like a cancer, thereby increasing the amount of virus produced and spread to the pups.

Species and strains of animals and microbes are constantly evolving in ways that help them better evade or fight each other. This explains why even wild animals do not always have perfect health—the animals may evolve, but the microbes are evolving too. How well our bodies can respond to new variants can depend on how quickly the microbes change, as well as on the size of the infection and how good our immune systems are more generally. Major changes can lead to pandemics, such as influenza in birds, pigs, and humans. Sometimes these major changes are because microbes can share genes, thereby spreading their ability to beat an animal's immune responses.

However, microbes and parasites do not actually want to *win* this arms race. Parasites will best survive and spread if they cause limited damage to their victims—only enough to get their own nourishment and allow themselves to be spread to others. If the microbes kill off their hosts too quickly, the animals will not have time to spread them to others before they die. If the microbes kill off all their potential victims, then they will die out too. Either outcome would be a somewhat pyrrhic victory. Microbes and parasites have often evolved alongside their original host species, often reaching levels where neither side wins outright. This means native animals may have some immunity that other animals lack, for example West African N'Dama cows have some resistance to Trypanosome parasites. As we shall see, it is when this balance is disrupted that major outbreaks can occur, for example when animals are introduced to microbes they have not met before or when their immune system is damaged by stress.

Animal medicine revisited

Despite the similarities among animals—in sickness and in health—the medical treatment different species receive can vary. A beloved pet—or human—may be generally expected to get better medical treatment than, say, most broiler chickens, brown rats, red-eyed tree frogs, or zebrafish. This difference is partly caused by—and partly causes—differences in how much veterinary scientists know about how to treat different animals. We know a lot more about some species (e.g. dogs) than we do about others (e.g. red-eyed tree frogs). However, scientists have probably collected more data about rats, mice, and zebrafish than about most other species.

Another difference is in the amount of money spent on different animals. Many individual farm animals are worth too little financially for commercial farmers to justify spending large amounts on their treatment. People are generally willing to pay more to treat their dogs, horses, or selves than on their rodents, finches, or fish. There are also big differences in how individual animals are treated. Some owners spend significant sums on their pets, including rats or birds, while others spend nothing on their cats. Some farmers can afford to give personal treatment to each individual animal, and some rare breeding animals are worth considerable amounts of money. Nevertheless, an animal's medical treatment generally does depend on its species.

The biggest difference is, unsurprisingly, between humans and non-humans. In the UK, veterinary medicines represent around

1 per cent of total drug sales, with human drugs comprising the rest; while the UK government provides free(ish) healthcare to humans worth over £100 billion annually, equivalent charity services for animals are worth far less than 1 per cent of that amount. Similarly, veterinary scientific research receives tiny grants relative to research on human diseases, and that limited funding is not equally spread over all species. Again, this does not mean that every human gets better treatment than every non-human, especially from an international perspective.

Another difference between anthropic and veterinary medicine is how clinicians relate to patients. Most non-human animals rarely present themselves for treatment voluntarily (although some seem to like their vets). They do not provide verbal histories of how they have been feeling recently (although some can use sign language, and all express some symptoms through their behaviour). They do not hand over money to pay for treatment (although, for farm animals, it is their 'productivity' that earns the money). They do not consent to treatment (although some laboratory animals can be trained to facilitate minor procedures). They do not follow prescriptions (although many can learn to self-medicate).

Domestic animals need their owners to do all these instead. Owners need to be able to identify signs of ill health, ensure their animals get treatment, and provide the time, effort, and money required, often while dealing with other financial pressures (or priorities), particularly in commercial farms, zoos, and laboratories. Owners also need to be emotionally able to place their animals' well-being above their own (e.g. in making difficult decisions about euthanasia and avoiding keeping the animal alive for the owner's benefit). This places a lot of responsibility on owners and can create difficulties in veterinary practice. Owners may seek veterinary treatment late or never, and may refuse to fund or comply with treatment recommendations. This can put the veterinarian in an impossible situation.

In many cultures, adult human patients are involved in deciding what treatment they do—or do not—receive. This is often considered a basic right of human patients. This concept seems meaningless for non-human patients who cannot understand medical information and would often prefer simply to escape from the hospital. Instead, veterinary science needs to aim at ensuring treatment is in the best interests of the patient. Veterinarians often seek permission to treat an animal because the latter is the owner's property, but, ethically, owners should not be allowed to make their animals suffer, especially when the health problems are due to how the owners have kept or treated those animals. Fortunately, healthier animals are usually preferable for their owners, but veterinarians can face conflicts where owners do not want what is best for their animal.

Even with caring owners, veterinary science has to cope with many challenges created by the differences between most human and veterinary patients. Veterinarians cannot use words to ask their patients what is wrong, or where it hurts, in order to better diagnose their problems. Veterinary scientists cannot ask them about their previous lifestyles or medical history in order to research the possible causes of their current conditions. Veterinarians cannot give animals information to help them understand their treatment and give them hope it will be effective. Veterinary patients may suffer because they can neither understand why they are being kept in a hospital and given unpleasant treatments nor look forward to their recovery. In some cases, this can make them resistant to treatment or even aggressive. Such situations can, of course, occur when treating some human patients too, but arguably less often.

Perhaps a more useful and precise comparison is between veterinary and paediatric anthropic medicine—accepting that this comparison may raise eyebrows among many medical researchers and practitioners. Babies also lack the ability to communicate their symptoms verbally or to understand medical advice. Until fairly recently, many people believed that babies felt less pain than adults, and so did not need pain-killers, but recent evidence suggests young animals (human or non-human) may actually experience pain *more* intensely, because their nerves have developed less. Babies rely on their parents to communicate with the clinicians; ensure treatment is in their best interests; and give good care at home. If parents fail in these roles, their preferences are hopefully outweighed by what is best for the child. The paediatric medical profession is a model for the relationships between veterinarians, owners, and patients.

Even in this comparison, two other ethical differences between anthropic and veterinary medicine are worth highlighting. The first is that veterinarians have to balance their duties to their patients with their responsibilities to humans, whereas little or nothing is generally said about anthropic doctors' duties to non-human animals. The second is that active euthanasia is a common and important part of veterinary work. Euthanasia is essentially killing an animal for his or her own good, where physical or psychological suffering cannot be avoided by other treatment options—or where those options are not available because of legal or financial restrictions. It is a vital part of veterinary medicine for all species, but it is emotionally demanding, especially in difficult and avoidable situations.

Chapter 3
Making illnesses better

Seeing what's wrong

An obvious part of veterinary science is making animals better when they are ill, injured, or disabled. And a first step to make animals better is usually to work out what is wrong for *that* animal. In doing so, veterinary science identifies what is abnormal—and what is normal—in their patients' bodies and behaviours.

Working out what is wrong is primarily for the benefit of the patient, in order to help determine what would be the best treatment. It can also help to predict how an animal's condition will improve or deteriorate. Working out what is wrong with one patient can also help other patients in the herd or species, who also need treatment or protection from similar conditions. Indeed, veterinary clinicians and researchers sometimes work out what is wrong in animals after they are dead, which certainly can only help other animals in the future. Veterinary scientists in practice must also try to work out what is wrong for patients' owners, who may well be affected by their animals' conditions such as their poor fertility, incontinence, or aggression, and who may want a particular outcome.

Owners and stockpersons also provide valuable information, which can be used alongside the veterinarians' personal observations and laboratory tests. Veterinarians need to find out about each animal's anatomy, physiology, and behaviour; and particularly about any changes over time. They need to be aware of contextual information about animals' demographics, environment, management, and lifestyle, especially where problems are more common in particular breeds (e.g. inherited disorders), ages (e.g. osteoarthritis), or husbandry systems (e.g. osteoporosis in caged hens). They also need to know whether other related or nearby animals are affected, and what controls are in place, especially for toxic, nutritional, infectious, or genetic disorders (e.g. quarantine, pasture management, and pre-mating tests).

Veterinarians use a variety of their senses to gain information about how animals' bodies are functioning (Figure 6). They can *see* if a bird is 'fluffed up' or a horse is lame; *hear* the coughing in a pig

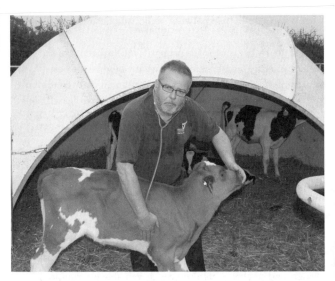

6. **The most important way of finding out what is wrong is by examination.**

shed; *feel* fat deposits or a fast pulse; or *smell* yeasty skin infections or ketones in a diabetic patient's breath. They could in theory even *taste* sugar in the urine of diabetic animals—but most veterinarians are probably not well enough paid for this. Observing animals from a distance helps in the assessment of their behaviour and demeanour, before they are too stressed by the human's proximity, perhaps trying to hide their illness because they see humans as predators. When it is safe to do so, veterinarians can then examine individuals from one end to the other, noting what is normal and abnormal. Observation and handling also allows us to judge how a patient responds to us: for example if a wild animal is apathetic to humans, this may suggest some serious illness.

In one sense, all veterinary work is scientific in that veterinarians in practice are collecting data to test hypotheses about their patients by using careful observations, laboratory techniques, and scientific theories to assess the form and function of particular body parts or biological processes. But veterinarians also need to consider each patient as an individual animal, and, for those kept in groups, as an interconnected herd or flock.

Looking deeper

Having made our initial observations, veterinary scientists can then perform various further tests. Providing food and water can help in assessing patients' appetite and thirst by seeing how keen they are to eat or drink. Pressing or moving particular body parts can help us to see where it hurts: for example lifting a cow's abdomen using a pole to see if they grunt in pain. Stimulating animals' senses can test their reflexes and see how their nerves, sense organs, and brain are functioning. For example, in some species shining a light into one eye would normally cause both pupils to constrict—if the lit-up pupil does not, it might suggest some problem in that eye's structure, retina, nerves, or musculature; if the *other* eye does not, it might suggest a problem in either eye or the nerves between them.

Veterinarians also look or listen within the animal. Veterinary surgeons can open the abdomen or a joint or use various 'scopes' to look inside eyeballs, ears, airways, intestines, joints, and abdomens. Veterinary imagers can show how different tissues—or substances put into the body—block, rebound, or emit a variety of electromagnetic and sonic waves (Figure 7). These can create images that may show abnormalities in the number, size, location, shape, margins, and appearance of tissues. For example, solid bones may stop X-rays but fractures let them through; and fluid-filled cysts rebound fewer ultrasound waves than solid tissue. Veterinarians also use the many fancy-sounding techniques employed in anthropic medicine such as CT, MRI, and PET scans.

Other tests can assess the function of particular organs. X-ray videos can show the movement of the throat when an animal swallows. Ultrasound videos can show the heart pumping

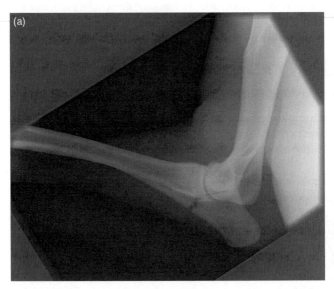

(a)

7. **Various tools create images of an animal's anatomy, physiology, or pathology including: (a) radiography.**

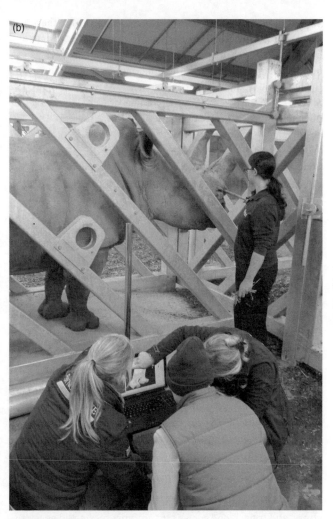

7. (b) thermography.

and even the movement of blood (e.g. through gaps in the heart or leaky heart valves). Radioactive atoms injected into a patient may be taken up by actively repairing bones, such as in bone cancers, fractures, and inflammation. Meters can detect the electrical signals of the heart muscles or nervous tissues. Pressure in the blood or an eyeball can be measured by seeing how much it resists force or how much force it takes to occlude an artery.

Samples such as faeces, urine, and swabs can be microscopically examined to identify microbes or parasites (or their eggs). Some microbes can be grown to see what species they are and what antibiotics might stop their growth (at least in a petri dish—which does not always mean they will be effective in the live animal). Other tests can identify parts of microbes' DNA or other molecules, and this can be especially useful for viruses, *Mycobacteria*, and anaerobic bacteria that are hard to grow outside of a body. For example, lumpy skin in cows may be due to a pox virus, herpes virus, or a fungus. Some of these are worse than others, and deciphering which one it is may require cells to be examined under a microscope. Sometimes these tests can only be done post-mortem, for example it is only by testing brain samples that veterinarians can reliably identify rabies or scrapie.

Veterinary scientists can look at tissue samples microscopically to see if the cells and structures are normal, often after staining them with particular dyes. If there are lots of inflammatory cells, this might suggest infection, injury, allergy, or that the body is fighting its own cells. If there are many strange or growing cells, this might suggest damage or cancer. Different levels or forms of blood cells may indicate anaemia, infections, stress, and some blood cancers. Examining sperm and eggs can show how well these are functioning. Looking at the cells that come from females' vaginas can show where they are in their reproductive cycle; or cells in their milk can indicate an infection in a cow's udder.

Veterinary scientists can measure the biological chemicals in bodily fluids in the blood, bladder, spinal cord, or joints to evaluate how well organs are functioning. Chemical tests can measure the concentrations of minerals, hormones, metabolic by-products, or chemicals produced by damaged cells to see if they are healthy. Looking to the future, as we improve our understanding of how diseases happen, we can identify new chemicals that give us earlier or more specific warnings when there is something wrong.

Veterinary scientists can also screen animals' genes. Genetic tests are likely to be of increasing importance in the future, particularly as veterinary science understands more about the genetics of normal domestic animals. Looking at animals' genes is not new—for half a century, scientists have identified abnormal, absent, or extra chromosomes (e.g. the additional X-chromosome associated with Klinefelter syndrome in cats). The key recent advances, as animals' genes are mapped (e.g. mice in 2002; and dogs in 2005), are in seeing if particular DNA sequences are lost, added, or altered; or if they are linked to specific diseases. As most diseases have both genetic and environmental parts, large numbers of each animal's genes may make them, and their relatives, more likely to get a particular disease. Screening for such increased risks is becoming more automated, faster, and cheaper.

Veterinarians can also increasingly use digital data such as GPS tracking of animals' movements (e.g. in following wild animals); pedometers to see changes in activity (e.g. during cows' reproductive cycles); microchips that can take biological measures; and machines to measure the electrical conductivity of milk to help detect signs of udder infections earlier. The expansion of telecommunications and Internet services may lead to greater use of home and field tests. Pigeon-fanciers can send faecal samples directly to laboratories, and dog owners can use home urine test kits and send photographs of the results for analysis. Looking forwards, there is a danger that owners could send samples or images to a laboratory without involving a veterinarian in the process. This leads to the risk of results being misinterpreted by owners who are without the necessary expertise; or by algorithms that miss other key signs needing to be taken into account.

Making it better

It is no good only working out what is wrong. The ultimate aim is to make it better. This might involve curing a health problem completely (e.g. surgery to remove a gut blockage) or slowing or reversing its development (e.g. stitching a wound to help it heal; or partially shrinking a tumour). Alternatively, treatments might reduce the unpleasant or harmful symptoms of a condition (e.g. pain-killers, anti-itch drugs, and anxiolytics). While it would be wonderful to be able to cure every disease, improving animals' quality of life by other means is an important part of veterinary

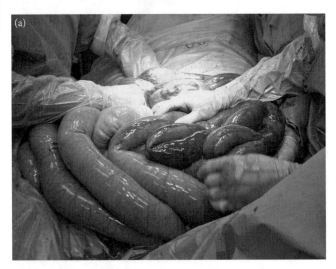

8. Surgery: (a) intestinal surgery for colic.

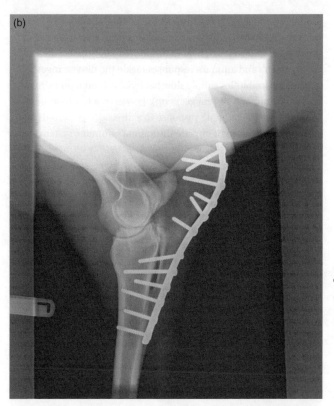

8. (b) orthopaedic surgery to repair the fracture shown in Figure 7(a).

medicine, in which there have been key recent advances (e.g. in
protocols for pain management). For example, chemotherapy may
kill off a cancer completely, but if not it may still slow its growth,
or even simply reduce its size so that it is less uncomfortable for
the animal to live with.

Treatments work in various ways. Some remove what is causing
the problem (e.g. an abscess or an object stuck in an animal's
airway, intestine, or bladder; Figure 8). Others replace part of
the body's function (e.g. giving insulin where the animal is not

producing enough). Many support the patient's body while it recovers by its own activities (e.g. holding a bone fracture or skin wound still so it can heal naturally). In many cases, the veterinarian's and animal's responses tackle the disease together (e.g. many antibiotics simply slow bacterial reproduction while the body's immune system gears up). However, a few treatments work *against* the animal's response to a disease (e.g. steroids and pain-killers are used to impede the animal's immune system, inflammatory processes, or pain responses).

Veterinary treatments tend to be of four broad kinds. *Drugs* may be applied directly to where they are needed (e.g. on the skin or in a joint) or so that they spread around the body (e.g. by injection into the blood or via the mouth or rectum). *Surgery* may remove or repair unhealthy tissues (e.g. from stitching up a minor wound to transplanting a kidney). *Advice* may change how owners care for their animals (e.g. by giving them more UV light, healthier diets, or therapy to overcome phobias). *Euthanasia* may end suffering where other treatments are not sufficiently likely to be beneficial. Multiple treatments are often combined in courses of care for each patient: for example a horse with colic may receive pain-killers and other drugs before and after surgery, and then require careful feeding to minimize further intestinal problems.

As in anthropic medicine, there are debates and scepticism around the value of therapies such as aromatherapy, homeopathy, and crystal healing. In particular, there is a debate currently as to whether veterinarians, belonging as they do to a science-based profession, should be allowed to prescribe homeopathic therapy even when the evidence suggests it is probably ineffective. Whatever the positive value of these alternative therapies, practitioners should ensure that they are, at worst, harmless. Any potentially toxic products should be avoided. And their use should never mean that animals are prevented from receiving proven, conventional treatments. They should therefore always be viewed as 'complementary medicine' not 'alternative medicine', and, where they are used, it should always be under veterinary guidance. Of greater concern are training methods that use painful punishment (e.g. electronic shock collars and whips) or severely restrict animals' movements (e.g. overly tight nosebands or *rollkur*), the use of which is often defended by outdated concepts like 'dominance theory'.

Recent decades have seen considerable advances in veterinary medicine, such as in the treatment of cancers, rabbit medicine, and improving animals' health on a herd level. Following anthropic medicine, veterinary scientists can expect to see advances in gene therapies, effectively programming animals' cells to be healthier; and in animal 'psychotherapy'. One recent idea is to use some microbes to fight others. For example, a bacteria called *Bdellovibrio bacteriovorus*, injected into the animals, could fight off *Salmonella* infections in chickens, conjunctivitis in cows, and *Shigella* bacteria in zebrafish, while also appearing to stimulate the animals' own immune systems.

However, there are also areas where veterinary medicine remains limited. For example, there are many treatments to reduce the pain or the progress of osteoarthritis, but no effective treatment in any species that effectively reverses the degeneration. As another example, large animal medicine is unable to humanely fix many broken legs because the animals need to stand on all four legs. Veterinary scientists also need to learn more about uncommon farm animals (e.g. ostriches) or pets (e.g. geckos) as they become more widely owned.

Making it worse

While treatments are meant to make animals better, they often come with risks of unintended side-effects. Some of these involve unpleasant treatment experiences. Surgery can cause pain; chemotherapy can cause nausea; handling and hospitalization can cause fear or loneliness. Some side-effects reduce the body's own responses. Anti-fever drugs effectively disrupt one of the body's natural methods for tackling infection; chemotherapeutic, hormonal, and anti-epileptic drugs may reduce white blood cell counts; sedatives may stop an animal coping with a scary situation. Other side-effects lead to additional health problems. Drugs can cause allergic reactions; hospitalization may cause the spread of microbes, potentially including resistant bacteria.

Other risks are less direct. Taking too long on too many tests to work out exactly what is wrong could delay the animal getting treatment. Spending too much money can mean owners are unable to afford more useful treatment later. Providing life-saving treatments or 'hospice-style' palliative care may actually mean that pets continue to suffer or wild animals are released only to subsequently starve. There have been some recent developments in veterinary palliative care which can reduce suffering in many patients. But such treatment options raise ethical questions when they cannot return animals to a full, normal, pain-free life. Arguably, it would be better for many patients to be given euthanasia.

Veterinarians can often give additional treatments to reduce the side-effects of treatments. Anti-nausea drugs can reduce the nausea from chemotherapy. Tranquillizers, anaesthesia, and pain-killers can reduce the stress and pain of handling and surgery (Figure 9). Recent years have seen tremendous advances in the understanding and willingness of veterinarians and farmers to use these drugs. Of course, drugs given to reduce side-effects may also cause their own side-effects. Anaesthesia can be unpleasant, and can lead to significant risk of later injury (e.g. horses may injure themselves when trying to get up while they are still wobbly on their feet). Some pain-killers can cause respiratory depression or kidney problems in individual patients. As such, treatments need to be chosen carefully and given correctly.

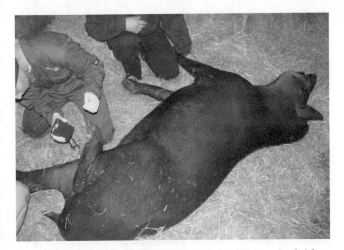

9. Anaesthesia can reduce the pain of surgery or the stress (and risks to humans), as in the case of this tapir.

Some treatments should, arguably, not be offered at all because the risks outweigh the benefits to the animal (although they may benefit the owner). The removal of claws, vocal cords, ears, or tails may make animals easier to keep or cosmetically more attractive, but they are painful and may prevent them from behaving normally. Some hormonal, medical, or surgical treatments may improve the reproductive or competitive performance of horses or farmed animals, but they may be painful or disrupt the animals' metabolism. Keeping suffering pets alive (slightly longer) may mean the owner can avoid (or, more accurately, delay) the bereavement, but it perpetuates the animal's suffering. Experimental treatments may advance veterinary medicine, but potentially at the expense of the individual patient's well-being. Some of these treatments might be considered illegal or unethical in some countries. However, all in all, veterinarians need to make their own assessments on what treatment will benefit the *patient* in each case.

Veterinarians need to balance the expected benefits with the potential harms, and know when intervening risks doing more harm than good. To do this, veterinarians need a solid basis of evidence from veterinary science to inform decisions. They need owners who are similarly empathetic and compassionate. They need to have enough information about the individual patient, how they might be expected to respond to each possible treatment, and how they might experience that treatment.

Getting it right

Scientific data still need to be interpreted into clinical decisions. Scientific studies focus on specific conditions within populations. But patients are all individuals. Different animals with similar symptoms may have different diseases. Neurological signs might mean epilepsy, a brain tumour, liver or kidney diseases, drug reactions, meningitis, or diseases like scrapie. Plus, the best treatment for each animal can depend on their age, body condition, other diseases, whether they are pregnant, personality, and so on. Clinicians need to balance competing concerns. For example, where pain-killers may sometimes risk kidney damage, veterinarians need to consider both the pain and the health of the kidneys, to determine whether the risks of kidney failure outweigh the pain they prevent for that patient (although this is not a reason not to give any pain-relief; rather, to choose carefully).

Veterinarians might tailor the treatments to individuals by careful dosing, especially for small, young, or ill animals who might be easily over-dosed. Chemotherapy drugs often have serious, dose-dependent, acute side-effects, so veterinary scientists may sometimes calculate doses using the patient's surface area. Anaesthetic drugs can be fatal if an animal is over-dosed; or they may leave the animal feeling the pain of surgery if under-dosed, so veterinary anaesthetists might give the drug slowly until the animal is sufficiently unconscious and then a lower dose that keeps them asleep—but not too deeply or for too long. Veterinarians might also measure blood concentrations or drug effects (e.g. heart rate) in real time, stopping when they reach the right doses or begin to see the occurrence of side-effects. On dairy farms, milk testing machines might be linked, via computers, to act *automatically* on those findings, for example in robotic feeding or milking systems.

Perhaps another way to tailor treatments in the future is to let animals choose their own medicines. Many wild animals seem to eat plants that may help against microbes or parasites; lame chickens appear to deliberately choose pain-killers; mice select drugs like diazepam in stressful situations; and many animals appear able to select foodstuffs to meet particular nutritional needs. Of course, veterinarians should always ensure the animals cannot choose toxic amounts of drugs or plants, and do not eat unbalanced diets that can cause nutritional deficiencies or excesses—the risks of this approach are clear from the commonness of diseases due to calcium deficiency, obesity, and metabolic problems.

Veterinary science also only gives us probabilistic data about populations—in practice, there can still be a lot of variation due to luck. A test might identify 90 per cent of cases of a disease, but in some cases it may get it wrong. Scientific studies might tell us that, statistically, 50 per cent of animals survive a given brain surgery, but that does not tell us whether a particular patient will. Veterinary decisions are only ever based on the probabilities of benefit and risks of harms. In retrospect, some correct choices at the time might then turn out badly for particular, unlucky animals. But unlucky outcomes do not mean that the decision was wrong.

Chapter 4
Making lives better

Back to the roots

As many wise non-veterinarians agree, prevention is better than cure. If a disease never occurs, we avoid all the suffering it can cause before it is recognized and treated. So a large amount of veterinary science involves trying to work out what causes problems, in order to tackle contributory factors and thus stop the disease process earlier in its tracks. Of particular importance for veterinary science are causes relating to the animals, their environments, genes, diets, prior conditions, and previous treatments.

Animals may get diseases directly from other animals. Infectious diseases may be spread through contact (e.g. ringworm and lice); sex (e.g. brucellosis and sexually transmitted tumours in dogs); or biting (e.g. rabies and facial tumours in Tasmanian devils). Animals may spread genetic diseases to their offspring (e.g. blood-clotting disorders and unhealthy body shapes) or pass on genes that make their offspring more susceptible to certain diseases in later life (e.g. scrapie and obesity). Veterinary science is also increasingly finding evidence that, as with humans, a pregnant mother being stressed, ill, poisoned, or starved may cause her offspring to be under-developed, ill, or pre-programmed to be at risk of various metabolic, psychological, or behavioural problems. Other diseases can be spread through the placenta or in milk (e.g. tuberculosis) or eggs (e.g. mycoplasmosis, which can cause respiratory disease, sinusitis, lameness, or death in poultry).

Some diseases are spread by invertebrate animals such as insects, ticks, snails, or molluscs. Ticks can spread *Borrelia* as they feed on dogs, horses, and humans (and other animals such as deer, rodents, birds, and lizards can also carry the ticks, although they are often not as badly affected by the disease). Mosquitoes may spread Rift Valley fever virus among cows, buffalo, goats, sheep, and camels in Sub-Saharan Africa, Madagascar, and the Arabian Peninsula. Sandflies can spread *Leishmania* among dogs, humans, and sometimes other animals. Tsetse flies and kissing bugs may spread Trypanosomes among humans, cows, and goats in Sub-Saharan Africa; and in humans, dogs, and opossums in the Americas. Invertebrates can also cause non-infectious diseases, and animals can be allergic to fleas or stings.

Animals may also get diseases or injuries from their environments. Environmental chemicals, hot or extreme weather conditions, and dangerous objects such as cars can cause burns, allergies, injuries, hyperthermia, and hypothermia. Threatening environments can lead to phobias or prolonged anxiety. Impoverished environments can lead to repetitive behaviours suggestive of mental health disorders, or conditions such as learned apathy. Some microbes can survive in water droplets in the air after they have been sneezed or coughed out of a carrier, then getting inhaled by other animals (so the medieval idea of miasmas was not so far wrong). Many gastroenteritis microbes or parasite eggs can survive for a period on dirty surfaces, bedding, housing, farm and hospital equipment, feed troughs or bowls—and on veterinarians themselves.

Some hardy microbes, such as parvoviruses, can even survive for a very long time after the infected animal has left, even surviving the effects of many disinfectants. Some other microbes live harmlessly in the environment, but can sometimes also infect animals. Tetanus bacteria live in the soil (and harmlessly in animal intestines or on our skin) but can accidentally enter an animal's body through a wound. *Aspergillus* fungi and botulism bacteria live in rotting plant matter but can be inhaled or their toxins eaten by cows, horses, dogs, or birds. *Aspergillus* can cause serious disease in seabirds who have never encountered the fungus at sea; while botulism can cause serious disease in ducks—with tens of thousands of birds killed (and maybe over a million during some outbreaks).

Animals' diets can be involved in causing a range of physical and mental health problems. Too much of the wrong food, or too little of the right food, for an animal's lifestyle can lead to obesity, starvation, nutritional deficiencies, or toxicities. Insufficient roughage can lead to poor digestion or to overgrown teeth that have not been eroded enough in animals whose teeth keep growing if they are not worn down by chewing. Food contaminated with other animals' faeces, urine, and abortion or placental fluids can spread harmful microbes. Young mammals (or humans of any age) may drink contaminated milk. Carnivores and omnivores may eat rodents or invertebrates with parasites in them—and herbivores may eat them by accident. Sometimes, farmers may even feed processed meat or bone to herbivores deliberately, which can create a risk of the spread of diseases such as scrapie and BSE—this is suggested to have caused the outbreak of BSE at the end of the last century.

Some diseases are effectively caused by other diseases. High stress levels may be linked to chronic viral infections. Viral respiratory disease may be followed by bacterial disease. And diseases that specifically reduce the effectiveness of an animal's immune system increase the risk that minor infections could cause full-blown illnesses. Furthermore, previous treatment for one problem can cause side-effects (as described in Chapter 2). In particular, continued behavioural therapy or training involving unpleasant or painful experiences may lead to animals becoming stressed or aggressive. When treating one problem, veterinarians need to avoid causing others (particularly if it is not a disease, but a normal behaviour such as barking).

It's complicated

Some problems have an obvious, simple, preventable cause, for example when a cat is hit by a car or a cow swallows something she shouldn't. But most diseases are not brought about by a single root cause. Many inherited diseases depend on the genes of both parents and their interaction with the environment. Many infectious diseases can be spread in multiple different ways. For example, equine arteritis virus (EAV) can be spread in the air, by sex, in the uterus, or via a contaminated environment. Furthermore, different individuals may be affected by the 'same' disease in various ways and to varying extents. Some might have a better immune response against an infection or be able to mobilize stored minerals during a nutritional deficiency.

Veterinary science often considers diseases to be caused by a combination of different factors. Anaphylactic shock can occur when the body is both over-sensitive to a particular chemical (e.g. bee venom or a drug) and has that chemical introduced into the body (e.g. through a bee sting or an injection). Nutritional deficiencies only occur when all sources of nutrition have proven insufficient for the animal's needs. Vitamin D deficiency may be due to both a lack of vitamin D in the diet *and* a lack of sunlight or artificial sources of UV that would help the animal make vitamin D. Obesity normally occurs when both an excess of calories is consumed and insufficient exercise is taken. Cancers may be caused by repeated exposure to carcinogenic chemicals or radiation. Indeed, it may be true to say that the majority of diseases are the result of the interactions between animals' bodies and their environment. Whether animals get ill can depend on multiple factors including interactions between the animals, the cause of the disease, and the animals' environment.

It is not always possible to predict which diseases animals might contract, and particularly difficult to predict in the case of an individual. But sometimes, by looking at populations, veterinary scientists can get an idea of which diseases are statistically likely to occur and how they might spread. Monitoring which animals have fallen ill or performing autopsies after they have died can indicate possible problems for other animals who have come into contact with them—either in life (as herds-mates or relatives) or after death (in food). Owners can be examined to look for possible causes of disease, and attempts can be made to prevent potential illness or to intervene early to minimize the effects. All of this surveillance requires the availability of a well-functioning veterinary infrastructure. And in detecting and preventing diseases in this way, a good veterinary industry provides important protection to human as well as non-human animals. In the future we may discover better ways to collect predictive data (e.g. by mining the data available in GPS telecommunications devices, from online shopping, and from medical data taken from across a broad spectrum of pet and stock owners) to predict the spread of disease.

It can be hard to know whether a potential risk factor is actually a cause of a disease or injury, or whether both are caused by something else. If an animal has arthritis and obesity, it may be unclear whether the obesity was caused by lack of exercise due to the arthritis; or the arthritis was caused by the pressure on the joints from the obesity; or both—or indeed if they were both caused by something else entirely. This logic is particularly important in genetics: groups of genes may code for multiple characteristics that therefore often come together. For example, Dalmatians' spots do not cause deafness, but their inherited set of genes can put them at 'risk' of both spottiness and deafness.

Consequently, some aspects of veterinary science consider all the factors that appear *associated* with an increased or decreased risk of an individual animal or a herd getting a disease. Large-scale studies of populations can show why and how diseases occur, and why their occurrence may vary across space, time, and situation. Such studies may become a major part of veterinary science, as digital data sources can be used alongside computer models to map and model complex land, populations, and social networks between animals. Other studies have been used to try to work out the chain of causation, for example by learning about animals' histories or subjecting individual animals to particular situations and seeing if a disease subsequently occurs. Sometimes it still remains unclear whether a risk factor causes a disease or is merely associated with it: for example in the relationship between excessive calorie intake, fatness, and Type II diabetes.

Every animal's well-being is important. But veterinary scientists often have to consider the health of all the animals within a herd, flock, wild population, or ecosystem. While it is impossible to keep every animal healthy all the time, veterinary science can reduce the overall risks and severity of all diseases for that group. This often requires veterinary scientists to carefully balance the risks of different diseases. For example, keeping dairy cows indoors on straw may reduce lameness but could lead to them getting some udder infections because they are in closer proximity to each other; there's greater risk of them standing on one another's teats; and dirtier surfaces can cause infection. Keeping hens in indoor cages may reduce their exposure to some diseases, but it puts them at risk of mental health disorders.

Choose your partners

One obvious way to prevent disease is to start with healthy animals in the first place. Such animals will hopefully remain relatively healthy—if they do not come into contact with other, infectious, animals—and should not pass on genetic and infectious diseases to each other. Farmers and owners can procure their animals from trustworthy breeders and farms that have been assessed and are free from particular diseases. Reciprocally, farmers may remove animals from an existing stock when they show signs of disease, or when they have been in contact with animals who do—either keeping them isolated from the rest of the herd or killing them. An example of this happening was in the large-scale culling programmes in the UK's eradication of a foot and mouth outbreak in 2001; or more recent efforts to control avian influenza.

Veterinary scientists can identify some unhealthy animals using the methods described in Chapter 3. Clinical examinations may spot signs of infectious or inherited diseases. However, animals may carry microbes or genes for a while before showing any sign of it—and some infected animals may never show signs at all. Sometimes, veterinary scientists therefore delay the introduction of new stock to other animals until they have had time to develop any potential, overt disease, effectively lengthening the clinical examination period. How long animals should be quarantined depends on the scientific information about how long it can take between an animal getting infected and then showing symptoms of the infection. This can vary from hours (e.g. some infections from cat bites); to many months or years (e.g. rabies and BSE); to indefinitely (e.g. some cows with tuberculosis).

However, even then, clinical examinations and quarantine will not pick up every disease. For example, cows might still carry the microbes that cause lumpy skin disease, tuberculosis, or brucellosis. So veterinary science has developed additional tests to detect unhealthiness in animals, often evaluating their genes or immune responses to molecules on the microbes (e.g. testing the immune response of cows to *Mycobacteria*; the DNA of cats for cystic kidney disease; the faeces of reptiles for parasites; and the brains of sheep for scrapie). Veterinarians can use these tests to check animals before they bring them onto the farm—and testing cows before moving them is a vital part of stopping the spread of tuberculosis. Veterinarians can use some of these tests after animals are euthanased or slaughtered—to decide whether the rest of their flock needs to be isolated and tested.

While gene therapy may still be largely a hope for the future, preventive genetic screening has a more imminent potential. Indeed, genetic testing can go beyond just screening for diseases, and help breeders to choose animals who will give their offspring the best chances of good health and productivity. Farmers and breeders can then breed dairy cows who are less prone to udder infections or lameness; sheep who are more resistant to common forms of scrapie; and outcrossed Dalmatians who avoid inherited bladder stones.

Breeders have always been able to use the 'genetic tests' of actually looking at animals and their relatives before deciding whether to breed them. Increasingly, veterinary scientists can also use big collections of data about animals' relatives and genetic profiling to help farmers choose healthier animals to buy or breed. The techniques are becoming increasingly affordable as the cost of genetic profiling decreases—costs have already been reduced by several orders of magnitude since the start of this century. Further research and commercial applications should bring significant developments in mapping animals' genes and linking genetic markers with economic and welfare characteristics.

The limitations in our ability to improve animal genetics will probably come not from veterinary science, but from the will of owners and society. Animals with infections or unhealthy genes may have other characteristics that their owners like, that improve their aesthetic appeal or reproductive, competitive, or productive performance. The snub faces that some dog owners find cute may leave the dogs struggling to breathe. Genetically programming animals to put lots of resources into growth (or breeding, egg laying, or milk production) may leave them with limited resources available for immune responses. As we saw, the gene sets and management methods that seem to put chickens or turkeys at greater risk of some health problems also make them grow quicker and more efficiently.

Healthy breeding therefore needs to be economically viable and culturally encouraged. Veterinary science can help would-be dog owners to choose pets in ways that support responsible breeding. Scientific assessments can help farmers to estimate the financial value of breeding from their available mating options (including using sperm from elsewhere) and to develop breeding strategies and programmes that take into account the mid- and long-term costs of ongoing diseases and the possible risks. The economic drivers are likely to be particularly important in developing countries, and issues of cost and intellectual property may need to be overcome. Fortunately, all breeders and farmers also have the more basic option of selecting good breeding animals whose offspring are likely to be healthier.

Cleanliness

Another way to reduce the spread of microbes or parasites is by removing, diluting, or killing them, by slowing their growth or by keeping animals away from them. They can be removed by cleaning, sewerage, water replacement, and ventilation. Their numbers can be diluted by flushing wounds with water, or keeping animals sufficiently spread out that microbe levels do not build up. They may be killed, slowed down, or made less viable by using disinfectants, high heat, pressure, refrigeration, preserving or drying them out, and some electromagnetic radiation (even sunlight can harm many microbes). They can be kept away from vulnerable animals by setting up barriers such as the use of sterile gloves and surgical gowns, using chemicals to repel or kill insects that spread diseases, or by ensuring animals avoid areas where particular microbes may be found.

Hygiene is especially important for people, vehicles, and equipment that move between animals. Each farm needs to be particularly careful to ensure that vehicles and people are cleaned and disinfected before they come onto the farm so that they do not bring in microbes—and do not spread the farm's own microbes elsewhere after they leave. Each hospital needs to ensure that the germs infecting one patient are not spread to the others nearby or in different wards. In fact, veterinarians themselves can spread microbes on their hands, clothes, equipment, and vehicles, as they travel around farms or perform surgery. Hygiene is also particularly important where animals are kept in large numbers and are ill or under stress, such as within hospitals, houses with lots of pets, some farms, and live animal markets.

Good hygiene requires following appropriate cleaning procedures. Microbes are not all beaten by the same hygiene methods. Parvoviruses can be resistant to many disinfectants. The misshapen proteins that cause scrapie and BSE may not be destroyed by heat or many disinfectants. Furthermore, some attempts at hygiene can actually spread disease: for example microbes can be spread on cleaning materials such as mops and muck-scrapers. Hygiene attempts are only as good as the weakest link—even if everybody else is scrupulously clean, it only takes one person to spread microbes.

At its extreme, the logic of hygiene might suggest isolating individual animals in completely sealed, sterile environments, as sometimes attempted in biosecure laboratories. Elsewhere, the more practical aim is to reduce microbes to low enough numbers that the animals' immune systems can fight them off. Good hygiene does not necessarily mean trying to create perfect sterility, but merely to reduce the amounts of microbes to defeatable levels. This is one place where the analogy of a battle works well: a small invasion can be beaten, but a large invading army of microbes can overwhelm the defences. How many microbes the animals can fight off depends on how healthy, immune, old, and stressed they are.

In fact, excessive sterility might be counter-productive. As described in Chapter 2, an animal's immune responses can develop through exposure to microbes, and without that exposure animals will not develop a good enough immune system to fight serious infections in the future. An animal whose system has never encountered a particular microbe (and successfully fought it off) may not be able to mount a good enough response when they get a serious infection. An excessive focus on creating sterile living conditions may also mean animals do not get enough beneficial microbes, particularly from their mother, which may also mean they lack enough of these allies to fight off less friendly infections. Furthermore, efforts to make environments sterile by making them impoverished could lead to stress for the animals, thereby reducing their immune systems' ability to respond to microbes and making them even more likely to succumb to future infections (Figure 10).

In addition, too much hygiene might have unintended consequences. There are some concerns that, as in humans, keeping surroundings and individuals too clean can be associated with allergies. This has been speculatively associated with a lack of beneficial bacteria, or it may be that under-stimulated immune

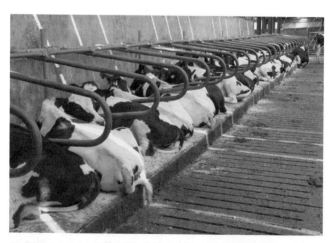

10. Keeping animals together in large numbers makes hygiene important, but it is not the only factor in designing environments for animals.

systems become over-reactive and fight against otherwise harmless chemicals in the food or environment. For example, some 'natural killer' white cells normally attack microbes or parasites but can also start to attack the body's cells. This may be less of a concern in non-human animals, who generally probably do encounter more dirt, either living on farms or going outside. Indeed, pets who are kept largely indoors do appear more prone to getting allergies (although some breeds seem more susceptible due to their genetic heritages). Sometimes exposure to microbes is a good thing.

Vaccination

Indeed, veterinary science does now tactically expose animals to microbes: in vaccination. Microbes like Newcastle disease viruses can be killed, modified, or broken into bits so they should not cause full-blown disease. They can then be sprayed on the animals, added to their water or food, or injected into them, so the animals' immune systems can develop better defences against them. Some microbes can also be altered to stimulate immune responses to *other* microbes without causing their diseases. For example, Newcastle disease virus can be used to carry molecules normally found on other viruses such as avian influenza, canine distemper, rabies, and Rift Valley fever, or even from bacteria such as *Borrelia*. These modified viruses can then be given to animals so they develop immunity against those molecules, and thereby against the other viruses or bacteria on which they are found.

In the future, veterinary science will have vaccinations made from tumours to boost animals' immune systems to fight cancer cells. For example, veterinarians may take tumour cells from the patient and re-inject their molecules into the animal to stimulate the patient's immunity, often combined with chemicals or the body's own immune cells that increase the body's response to them. Veterinary scientists might also modify viruses so that they have tumour cell molecules on their surfaces. In the USA and Europe, veterinarians have recently developed a way to inject (human) cancer-related DNA into dogs, which stimulates their immune system to fight melanoma cells—although clinical successes are not perfect, and there is uncertainty as to how much these treatments really do affect the animals' immune responses.

Veterinary scientists want to make sure that vaccinated animals mount strong immune responses to the molecules. Vaccine injections often contain other chemicals that stimulate the animal's immune system. Multiple vaccines can give animals' immune systems more chances to develop and maintain their immunity. Veterinarians try not to vaccinate animals when they are ill as their immune systems may already be busy; they also avoid vaccinating unweaned mammals when their mother's antibodies from her milk may fight the microbes off without the animal's own immune system having to do anything. However, waiting too long after the maternal antibodies have diminished could leave the animal with no immunity—at a time when they need to be out learning about the world to avoid mental health problems. So veterinarians often have to give multiple, carefully timed boosters over several weeks to ensure some of them work.

Individual animals will each benefit from being vaccinated against common diseases that they might encounter. For example, in many countries dogs may come across distemper, parvovirus, and rabies viruses, and vaccination can help them avoid fatal infections. However, the main benefit of vaccination is in reducing the levels of disease in a whole population—this 'herd' then becomes healthier overall. If enough animals are sufficiently immune to a disease, then this can mean the microbes cannot spread between animals quickly enough and, as victims die or recover, the microbes themselves also then die out. When enough animals are vaccinated this can eradicate diseases—as has been achieved for cattle plague and, in many countries, rabies.

However, vaccination is not risk-free. Like other medicines, it has potential side-effects. Vaccines are effectively deliberate infections and can still cause some—hopefully minor—illnesses (e.g. cats given 'flu' viruses may then have brief flu symptoms). Some vaccine injections (e.g. against rabies and the feline leukaemia virus) might also lead to a tiny percentage—one per several thousand—of animals forming a cancer (perhaps depending on the patient's genes). Such minor risks have caused serious anxiety about vaccination among some pet owners (and some children's parents regarding combined measles vaccinations). Some people may therefore fail to have their animals vaccinated, putting them at greater risk of getting preventable and fatal infectious diseases. Veterinarians need to balance the risks rationally to ensure animals get the right vaccines often enough to ensure they can develop adequate immune responses to the microbes they are likely to meet.

Another risk of vaccinations is that they might interfere with the tests used to screen animals. As described in Chapter 3, our tests often involve assessing an animal's immune response to a microbe. A strong immune response suggests they have met that microbe, and so might be infected. However, animals may show a similar immune response to a vaccine—without thereby becoming infected. So vaccinating animals may make tests less reliable at identifying real infections. This is one reason against vaccinating cows against tuberculosis: it reduces our ability to test cows before moving them. Fortunately, recent studies suggest that there may soon be a test that can distinguish vaccinated from infected cows, although the research and development of a field-ready product needs speeding up.

Another concern with vaccinations is that they may not always be effective. Some microbes come in such a variety, with different chemicals, that making animals immune to a small subset does not prevent them being infected by other, slightly different, types. Other microbes may 'evolve' into strains whose molecules are somewhat different to those used in existing vaccines. Sometimes, this can mean that the animal's immune system does not recognize the new chemicals, and thus no longer fights off those microbes. This is yet another 'arms race', this time between the microbes and the pharmaceutical companies. This means vaccines need to be kept up to date to reflect the strains found in the particular geographical location in which they are used. For example, in recent years, there have been new vaccine strains for horse influenza and dog Leptospirosis (which can cause kidney or liver failure).

Treating diseases before they occur

Another way to prevent illnesses is to treat their causes before they get bad enough to represent major problems. Vitamin supplements may head off mild deficiencies. Washing hooves with antiseptics can kill microbes that might otherwise build up on the skin. Drugs can kill worms, lice, and fleas before their numbers build up. Antibiotics may prevent infections, if there is a risk that an operation has introduced microbes into an animal's wound or body cavities, or when an animal has been exposed to infected animals. Historically some farmers have also given low doses of antibiotics to cows, pigs, chickens, turkeys, and fish, to deal with ongoing infections on farms. This is now considered contrary to good practice and is decreasing in many countries due to human health concerns regarding antibiotic resistance.

Altering animals' bodies can also reduce some risks of later illnesses or injuries. Many pets are neutered, which can mean they avoid fatal womb infections and cancers. Many farm animals have parts of their bodies removed or shortened, such as their tails, beaks, teeth, horns, or skin (e.g. around their buttocks) with the intention of preventing them from suffering or causing injury to other members of their group. A good example is tail docking. For pigs, it is aimed at preventing injuries from pigs biting one another's tails. For cows, it is argued that it helps avoid udder infections—although there is little evidence it helps (arguably it is more to avoid farmers being flicked in the face during milking). For sheep, it may help avoid faeces building up in their wool that can then get infested with damaging maggots. For dogs, it was originally done to prevent tail injuries when working dogs chased through the undergrowth, but it can now be carried out as a practice that has become cosmetic 'plastic surgery' as part of the 'look' of that breed.

Some of these interventions are illegal in some countries, but even legal operations are controversial. Veterinarians have a responsibility to consider whether such treatments really will be beneficial for their patients: the welfare benefit to each animal needs to be greater than that of having the body part remain intact. On the one hand, the procedures often involve painful surgery, particularly when done to very young animals without anaesthetic or painkillers, and they may interfere with the animals' behaviour. On the other hand, veterinarians may be nervous about leaving pigs undocked on farms that routinely dock their piglets' tails, in case they are proven wrong and there is a catastrophic result for those pigs.

There are often better ways to prevent problems, but these can often be perceived as coming at an additional cost. Low-grade infections might occur more often when farms have larger numbers of animals living close together, poorer hygiene, or where animals are stressed by a lack of space and impoverished environments. Similarly, tail-biting can occur more often in farms with preventable health problems, poor diets, or barren environments (e.g. bare, slatted floors where pigs are not given enough space to explore, root, and chew). If a farmer can rely on the low-level use of antibiotics or being able to tail dock their pigs, arguably they have less of a reason to carefully select their animals, or to maintain a hygienic and healthy environment, giving their pigs, for example, better environments and enough straw, which thereby also improves their mental health. However, if a veterinarian refuses to allow treatments such as tail docking this creates a risk that animals could still suffer from being kept in the poor conditions *as well as* from the consequences of, not having their tails docked in those circumstances.

Rightly, this dilemma makes such treatments controversial. Where science has found practical ways to reduce risk factors for such diseases, farmers need support to make any necessary changes and not allow poor farming practices to continue. But animals should not be left to suffer catastrophic injuries or illnesses where the problems cannot be—or perhaps, more often, simply are not yet being—reliably eliminated or sufficiently reduced. This dilemma leads to compromises such as an EU law that might ban tail docking except as a last resort when other methods have been tried and have not reduced tail-biting satisfactorily. This loophole has allowed tail docking to remain common (albeit banned completely in a few member countries such as Sweden, Lithuania, and Finland—where around 1 to 2.5 per cent of pigs do suffer from having their tails bitten). But, rather than changing the animals to fit a particular farming system, veterinary science aims to re-design our farming environments to fit the animals.

Good care

In general, the most important way to prevent diseases is to ensure that animals get the right care to keep them healthy. Many conditions are caused by an animal's diet, environment, and company, so how they are kept is probably the key determinant of whether they stay healthy. Good care should also give animals the resources they need to deal with health problems and other challenges. Thus, the best way to keep animals generally healthy is to keep them generally well cared for. The best way to avoid vitamin D deficiency is simply to give reptiles the right (natural or artificial) lighting and diet. The best way to avoid mental health problems is to provide stable, pleasant environments and beneficial companionship.

A good diet is essential for all animals. All animals need to be able to avoid suffering excessive hunger and thirst, to maintain a healthy body, and to meet additional demands such as growth, reproduction, milk production, and exercise. Animals also need to avoid taking in nutritional excess (i.e. owners can avoid obesity by ensuring there are not more calories going into the animal than are being used up). Diets need to include the right food for efficient, healthy digestion (which will support beneficial intestinal microbes) and they need to be provided in the right way. Animals should be fed in a way that is in line with their natural eating behaviours, such as being able to forage and chew, in order to protect their dental, mental, and general health. Similarly, animals need to be provided with water in ways suited to their needs (e.g. to be able to drink it, to take it in from foliage, or to absorb it through the skin). And of course all diets need to be provided without large amounts of toxins or harmful microbes.

All animals also need a suitable environment that is safe, comfortable, clean, and hygienic—not too sterile but not overly dull either (Figure 11). The environment should allow animals to enjoyably use their senses, to rest comfortably, and to move, exercise, and play in ways that maintain their physical and mental health. Environments need to be large enough in all three dimensions, sufficiently complex, and predictable enough to give animals adequate stimulation without making them scared. Animals need to be able to control their environment, and have an appropriate range of safe options from which they can choose. For example, reptiles should be given a range of environmental temperatures and humidity across which they can move, according to their changing needs; and robotic parlours can reduce stress by allowing the cows to come and be milked as often as they need to be during the day. The very acts of choice and control can themselves be helpful in allowing animals to cope with challenges.

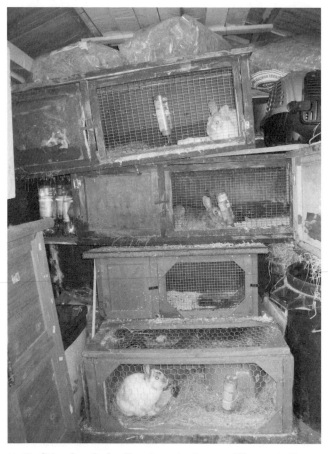

11. Traditional methods of keeping animals may well be unsuitable, as for these rabbits in hutches.

Animals also need the right company. Some species are generally social, and rarely choose to be alone. Such animals need positive and consistent company to help them control their temperature, deter flies, and groom one another. Good companionship may not only prevent the stress of isolation, but may also provide a necessary buffer against other challenges and increase resilience. Animals also need to avoid unsuitable company that may cause injuries, spread disease, cause unwanted pregnancies, prevent animals getting to resources they need, or cause stress. Animals should not be kept at overly high population densities. In addition, some animals are largely solitary (except perhaps for mating and childcare), such as many reptiles, hamsters, and small cats, and these should be able to avoid the contact of other animals.

Humans provide a separate source of company for some domestic animals. Some pets are very attached to their owners or their family, and can become significantly anxious when separated or left alone. Human caregivers can also provide some of the benefits of company, although they are not a replacement for the company of an animal's own species. Humans can also provide beneficial opportunities for exercise, stimulation, and learning. However, humans should avoiding causing their animals injury, pain, or fear, particularly when training animals or keeping animals who are naturally scared of humans. Even for domesticated animals, it is important to make sure young animals meet humans in pleasant ways, so they get used to them and learn to enjoy their company.

Indeed, domestic animals' health is particularly dependent on their owners, who determine their environments and genetics. Breeders decide which animals breed with whom. Owners decide how animals are kept, what they eat, and which other animals they meet. Many crucial aspects of preventing disease involve ensuring animals have what they need and are not overly stressed. So, in many ways, preventing disease in domestic animals is often just a matter of choosing the right animals to breed and then simply caring for them well. Conversely, where exotic animals are becoming more popular, veterinary science can learn more about their needs in order to better advise their owners. For wild animals, preventing disease may be best achieved by leaving them alone, an idea considered further in Chapter 6.

This means that improving animals' health is often a matter of improving owners' behaviour. For many owners, this is achieved by learning more about veterinary science—once they understand what their animals need, they can try to provide it. Other owners may need additional support or encouragement to motivate them, particularly when they need to change their behaviour significantly or spend a lot more of their time or money. Veterinary science can also identify ways in which helping animals may well pay for itself in commercial settings, through leading to better productivity—although this still requires farmers to have the necessary cash-flow for investment. Similarly, veterinarians can encourage owners to get health insurance for their animals—or not to get animals they cannot afford.

Veterinary science can help to inform psychological and cultural aspects that affect the care that owners give to their animals. Psychologically, veterinarians can give owners reminders to give their animals flea control, or weigh their animals to prompt them to change their diet or exercise, or help them understand that pets do not need to have had a litter before being neutered. Similarly, veterinary science can help farmers appreciate the value of having (fewer) productive animals rather than (more) skinny and unproductive ones. These changes need to be done in ways that respect the animals' cultural value, for example among some traditional African groups where cattle ownership can be related to status, marriage, funeral rites, traditional laws and societal value systems, and which ensure that, after droughts or famines, the farmer and animals have the best chance of surviving to better times. It can also draw on ideas of naturalness, for example to encourage giving dairy cows pasture, which can improve their wellbeing, and reduce their risks of lameness, mastitis and some metabolic and infection diseases.

Chapter 5
Diseases across species

Comparative medicine

Some microbes are not very picky about where they live. Cattle plague virus could also infect antelopes, buffalo, deer, giraffes, wildebeests, and warthogs. Canine distemper can spread to bears, civets, elephants, ferrets, mink, otters, raccoons, pandas, lions, hyenas, jackals, seals, and Japanese monkeys. 'Bovine' tuberculosis can infect cows, goats, sheep, African buffalo, bison, deer, elk, pigs, horses, dogs, cats, badgers, rabbits, guinea pigs, primates, brushtail possums, and primates; and its bacterial ancestors probably came from humans in the first place. Various types of influenza can infect ducks, chickens, turkeys, humans, pigs, horses, seals, whales, mink, cats, and bats. West Nile virus can infect species from humans and horses to alligators and geese. Rabies can affect many mammals and birds. *Salmonella* can possibly infect all mammals, birds, and reptiles—and even some plants. *Leishmania* can infect dogs, rats, raccoons, cows, pigs, and humans. *Toxoplasma* can reproduce in cats, but can also infest humans, goats, sheep, pigs, mice, rats, dolphins, manatees, sea otters, seals, sea lions, pandas, polar bears, and birds. Indeed, many parasites live in one animal for their early lives and another in a later stage.

This multi-way spread of microbes and parasites across species is concerning for several reasons. It means they can have a greater impact on more animals—of any species—who can get infected. It enlarges our 'herd' of animals through which microbes may spread. Separated populations of one species might have microbes or parasites spread between them via another species. Or one species in which the microbes do not survive for long (or whom it nearly wipes out) might contract them from another species with which they are in contact. Thus, some animals might get infected with microbes that they would not otherwise encounter. This can mean that the new species are naive to the microbe, and thus have limited immunity. Plus, as microbes spread across species, they might change in ways that make them more dangerous for other species. For example, flu virus strains might change genetically as they spread through wild birds, poultry, pigs, and humans.

Some microbes are relatively harmless for the species with which they have co-evolved, but fatal when they infect another species who have not developed such immunity. Grey squirrels may be relatively immune to the pox virus that can seriously harm red squirrels. Many birds may get Newcastle disease with limited effects, but it can cause significant illness when it infects domestic chickens. Bordetella, which causes respiratory disease in birds and mammals (it causes whooping cough in humans), is relatively harmless for rabbits but can be fatal for guinea pigs. There are lots of different influenza viruses that can infect birds, but many probably cannot pass to humans or are not that bad if they do. Rabies is almost always fatal in mammal species, but some bats may be able to tolerate it. Many reptiles have *Salmonella* on them, which seems harmless (or might perhaps even be beneficial) for them—but which might cause serious gastroenteritis for humans. There might also be some cross-species spread of beneficial microbes: owners share skin bacteria with their pets.

Of particular concern—for humans—are diseases that humans can get from other species (Box 12). Various estimates suggest that around 60 per cent of human disease microbes can infect other animals. Many of these are not new. Humans and animals have

Box 12 Selected disease-causing organisms shared by humans and other animals

Viruses

Hendra
Influenza
Nipah
Rabies
Rift Valley fever
West Nile
Zika

Bacteria

Mycobacterium bovis (bovine tuberculosis)
Brucella
Leptospira (Weil's disease)
Salmonella
Escherichia coli (*E. coli*)
Yersinia pestis (bubonic plague)

Fungi

Arthrodermataceae (ringworm)
Cryptococcus
Emmonsia parva
Geomyces destructans (white nose syndrome)
Histoplasma capsulatum (histoplasmosis)
Lacazia loboi (Lobo's disease)
Sporothrix schenckii

Parasites

Anisakis simplex
Borrelia (Lyme disease)
Leishmania

(continued)

Box 12 Continued

Schistosomes
Taenia solium (cysticercosis and taeniasis)
Toxoplasma
Trichinella
Trypanosomes (sleeping sickness and Chagas disease)

long shared diseases such as bubonic plague, leishmaniasis, tuberculosis, and brucellosis, and parasites such as tapeworms. Even measles may have come from cattle plague viruses that got into humans several thousand years ago. However, maybe 75 per cent of 'new' human diseases are found in other species. Plus, several more recent human diseases also have *suspected* links with other species who can get similar infections (e.g. bushmeat primates can get diseases similar to HIV and Ebola; and bats and civets have viruses similar to SARS and MERS). The future may see even more diseases spread across species, perhaps particularly of viruses, fungal infections, and lifestyle-related conditions.

Unsurprisingly, humans share diseases with monkeys and apes because all primates are closely related. Equally unsurprisingly, humans may share diseases with domestic animals that get eaten or live in human homes. But humans theoretically might share microbes with almost any species. Bats and rodents are of particular interest as sources of infection for other species, for example fruit-eating Old World bats are linked to rabies, Hendra, and Nipah viruses. It is unclear why. It may be that their different immune systems, high body temperatures, or hibernation patterns mean they are good at incubating viruses. Or it may be more simply because bats and rodents represent around 60 per cent of mammal species and are widespread; that bats can fly over large distances; and that many rodents colonize urban areas. However, the fact that bats can be linked to many types of virus does not necessarily mean they are important in spreading all of them.

It may be unhelpful to think of microbes as spreading one-way from non-human to human animals. Humans can spread most human diseases to one another (and the same applies for other animals). Humans can also give microbes and parasites to other species, including influenza, measles, *Salmonella*, *Campylobacter*, and tapeworms. Bovine tuberculosis, canine hepatitis, and some tapeworms probably all came from humans in the first place. Plus, most microbes *of course* come from another species at some point—discounting the discredited idea of spontaneous generation—and, with several million species of animals, it is statistically inevitable that lots of human diseases will have come from other species. A better way of looking at the situation is that humans and other animals *share* diseases due to our shared biologies and environments. When it comes to health, it can be useful to consider all animals as part of a wider 'herd'—human and non-human, domestic and wild.

Within this wider herd, microbes and parasites may be spread between animals of different species in the various ways described in Chapter 4 (except from parents to offspring). In particular, one animal may eat infected, infested, or contaminated meat, eggs, or milk; come into direct contact with another species or its environment; or consume another species' faeces. In many ways, human civilization seems set up to facilitate such a spread: humans cohabit with pets, eat many animals, feed some animals to others, and live near wildlife whose diseases may spill over to domestic animals or humans. The risks of subsequent infection then also depend on an animal's ability to fight infection—which will depend on their previous exposure, general health, immune system, and degree of stress. Fortunately, veterinary science can help us to use methods described in Chapter 4 to reduce the spread of microbes across species.

Minding the gap

Veterinarians, owners, and other public health workers can try to reduce the spread of microbes across species. One common method is to kill one species to protect another—usually killing wildlife to protect domestic animals (e.g. badgers or possums in areas where many cows have tuberculosis) or humans (e.g. rats, cats, and dogs in bubonic plague outbreaks); or killing domestic animals to protect humans (e.g. dogs to control rabies; or chickens to manage avian influenza outbreaks). Some schemes kill large numbers of animals. Millions of chickens have been killed (and billions of dollars spent) trying to reduce the risk of H5N1 avian influenza. Similarly, tackling Nipah controversially involved killing thousands of pigs and almost destroying the Malaysian pig industry.

Schemes that kill only suffering animals (e.g. rabid dogs) also effectively provide valuable euthanasia. More indiscriminate killing is harder to justify, particularly as such schemes are ultimately generally doomed to failure if the causes of the diseases remain. Except where island populations are completely exterminated, infections can re-appear when any remaining animals breed, nearby animals move, or farmers re-populate their sheds. Schemes are also hard to justify if they use inhumane methods such as poisoning, inaccurate shooting, or 'passive' killing by placing animals in over-populated shelters to die from stress, starvation, or infectious disease. It is better to ensure there are stable populations of healthy animals, for example through neutering and vaccination.

In some cases, killing animals can have the unintended and paradoxical side-effect of actually spreading more disease. In England in 2001, a foot and mouth disease outbreak was halted by killing many cows, sheep, and pigs. Afterwards, farms restocked by buying cows from elsewhere in the country. However, where these cows were infected with tuberculosis, this was thereby spread to new areas. Faced with widespread tuberculosis, the government has killed thousands of badgers, although the science behind this decision is at best ambiguous in deciding whether this would help or only worsen the problem. The available science suggests killing may, at least in some cases, actually spread tuberculosis, by disturbing the badgers' family and social units so that the badgers move around more. Killing badgers may also distract from efforts to control the disease in cows.

Another method is simply to keep species separate. Laboratories studying animal diseases maintain strict protocols to stop microbes or infected animals escaping. Some pet owners also separate themselves from their pets by abandoning them or giving them up when they get pregnant, in fear of miscarriages from diseases such as toxoplasmosis—rather than employing less extreme ways to avoid infection such as washing their hands. This means they forgo the benefits of pet ownership, such as potentially lower risks of allergies and skin problems in children whose mothers lived with dogs during their pregnancies. Farm management can limit contact between wild and domestic animals on farms or in stressful live markets. Public policy can make human habitats less attractive to other animals (e.g. through avoiding extensive open urban rubbish tips). Land management can minimize habitat destruction and disruption that makes animals move around and avoid encroachments on wild ecosystems that bring humans and domestic animals into closer proximity to wildlife.

Animals can also be kept nutritionally separate. Many countries have banned the feeding of meat products to farm animals, and some people may become vegan or make their pets vegan to avoid infections from meat, milk, and eggs (although this is unhealthy for properly carnivorous species such as cats). Recently, as BSE is partially forgotten, there may be a temptation to relax the restrictions to feed meat by-products to some farm animals (particularly pigs and poultry), in order to improve profitability.

The difficulty is knowing whether this is safe—any new diseases may, like BSE, build up until it is too late. As considered in Chapter 4, prevention is better than cure—and sometimes that means being cautious where the risks are uncertain.

Meat can also be processed in ways that reduce the spread of toxins, microbes, and parasites. Animals can be checked before they are slaughtered (although bushmeat bypasses such checks) or afterwards in mini-autopsies that examine the animals (e.g. looking for larval cysts or tubercles); their immune responses can be tested (e.g. counting white blood cells in milk); or they can be tested for the microbes (e.g. *Listeria*, which can cause neurological problems and miscarriage). Butchery can remove body parts that might contain particular microbes, such as brains and lymph nodes to reduce the risk of BSE and tuberculosis. Slaughterhouses can be kept clean to avoid microbes spreading from animals' intestines and skin onto the meat. Food processors can kill microbes and parasites by cooking, pasteurizing, or irradiating meat, eggs, or milk before they are eaten by animals, or at least they can slow the growth of the microbes and parasites by freezing, refrigerating, and preserving methods.

It is also important simply to ensure good hygiene in contact between species, by reducing the risks of one species eating or inhaling others' faeces and (for humans) by washing hands after contact with animals, particularly after contact with their bodily fluids or any uncooked meat. This may be particularly important for veterinarians treating animals who might have infections such as influenza or Hendra viruses, or for people whose immune systems are impaired for the reasons noted in Chapter 2. Hygiene can also reduce the spread of microbes from humans to other animals: for example people with flu symptoms should generally avoid unnecessary contact with ferrets, pigs, or birds.

Most importantly, species-crossing diseases can be prevented like other diseases, using the methods described in Chapter 4. Animals should be kept sufficiently clean, well-nourished, well-ventilated, and unstressed. They can be vaccinated against common diseases that infect other species, for example by inoculating hens against *Salmonella* to protect people who eat their eggs. Their health can be carefully monitored to identify emerging diseases in individuals, herds, and populations. When diseases do occur, veterinarians can recognize and treat those individuals quickly. Farmers and governments can keep good records of how animals are moved, in order to trace outbreaks back to their sources and identify other animals who might be at risk. Healthy animals should present less risk to other species.

Concerns about animal diseases might suggest all animals should be indoors and completely sterile. However, when overdone, this can be a risky strategy. First, if these are impoverished environments, then the stress caused may actually suppress the animals' immune systems. Second, their immunity to microbes can be improved by having encountered other microbes before, and having harmless or helpful microbes on their skin, in their airways, and in their intestines. So making animals' environments too sterile may actually make them more susceptible to microbes. They may have fewer infections in the short-term, but eventually microbes could spread and the animals might have little defence against them.

Rabies provides a good example of how improving health needs careful, clever, comprehensive, and collaborative thought. Major public health programmes have managed to eradicate rabies from some countries, but in many—often poor—countries, it is still common, particularly among dog populations. Tackling rabies needs a major, coordinated effort. This needs to focus on vaccinating dogs and wildlife against the disease. Better care needs to be provided for community dogs, neutering them to manage numbers—and not by simply killing them, which can just mean other dogs then move into the area. Humans need to be educated about the signs of disease in dog behaviour. The underlying issues of poverty and lack of infrastructure, and human and veterinary medical care need to be tackled. This will mean further veterinary scientific studies to better understand the ecology of community dogs, to develop effective and safe oral vaccines, to develop non-surgical methods to neuter animals, and to study the level and spread of the microbes.

Superbugs

Chapter 2 described how microbes may adapt in ways that evade animals' immune systems. Chapter 4 showed how this can put them in an arms race with new vaccines. In similar ways, microbes and parasites can also adapt to cope with drugs used to treat infections, so that they become resistant to those drugs. Such drugs may kill off susceptible microbes but allow more resistant microbes to survive. Consequently, there is now evidence of resistance to drugs among many parasites such as worms and Trypanosomes, some viruses, and bacteria such as *Campylobacter*, *E. coli*, *Salmonella*, *Clostridium*, and, most famously, *Staphylococcus aureus*—which may become resistant to drugs including methicillin (i.e. methicillin-resistant *Staph. aureus*, or MRSA).

The use of multiple drugs can mean that microbes and parasites become resistant to all those drugs, risking that veterinarians and anthropic medics run out of ways to treat ill humans or non-human animals. Resistant microbes might also spread between animals, in the ways described in Chapter 4, including from humans to other species and vice versa. As they reproduce, they pass on their genes that confer such resistance. Some microbes can also share their genes with others. These processes can lead to bacteria that are resistant to many drugs such as MRSA and *Clostridium difficile*.

This evolution can happen quickly—some bacteria became resistant to penicillin within months of its release onto the market. Exactly how quickly depends on several factors. Microbes and parasites may develop resistance quicker if drugs are used frequently. They may spread resistant genes faster if microbes are generally spread through poor hygiene or large animal groups. Both processes might happen faster if drugs are used in ways that allow some microbes to survive, for example at low doses or for short courses, or when the patient's own immune system is impaired. It is probably impossible to stop the development of resistance (unless society stops using such drugs altogether), but it may be possible to slow the increase in resistance by changing how animals are cared for, and how drugs are prescribed and used. Hopefully it can be slowed down enough to give us time to find new antibiotics—to keep us just ahead in the arms race.

The resistance to our current drugs is a strong driver to look for new drugs to which microbes and parasites are still naive. However, scientists have found very few new antibiotics for the last half-century. Researchers are currently looking at some potential sources of new drugs, such as chemicals in Tasmanian devils' milk, Komodo dragons' blood, and human noses. Others are re-examining older methods such as using a mixture of cow bile, wine, and garlic that was described in the Anglo-Saxon *Leech Book*, which appeared to kill MRSA in mice who had been given chronic, infected wounds. However, this pharmacological arms race is currently being won by the microbes. Even many of the relatively new drugs—often restricted to human use—already have encountered resistance in bacteria such *E. coli* and *Proteus* in south Europe. Global efforts need to focus on slowing the development of resistance.

The key battleground in the war against resistance is in hospitals, which bring together many ill patients, many on long-term drugs that suppress their immune systems (e.g. to treat cancer). All patients should get the drugs that they need, but these need to be the right drugs, getting to the right part of the body, at the right dose, for the right length of time. Before using drugs, clinicians should try to perform the right tests to diagnose the problem, identify the microbes, and determine whether those microbes are resistant to particular drugs (except in emergencies). Plus, in fact, many patients actually do not need anti-microbials at all, particularly for many acute gastrointestinal, respiratory, urinary, skin, and viral cases, and after sterile surgery. Most importantly, hospitals need to avoid spreading microbes between patients through poor hygiene. These principles apply to all medical hospitals—anthropic and veterinary.

Another battleground is on farms that contain large numbers of animals, cause them stress, and use long-term, low doses of drugs to reduce illnesses (and to promote growth, perhaps by preventing lots of low-grade infections). Resistant *E. coli* were found in farm animals and meat in China in 2015; and in a worker and several animals in a pet shop in 2016. Just as in hospitals, ill animals on farms should get the drugs they need to avoid them suffering (and this ethical duty applies on organic farms as much as others). The desire to reduce the use of antibiotics should not prevent ill animals getting the antibiotics they need. But farms should be well-run so that *routine* antibiotics are not needed, and never used simply to increase growth and profit. Fortunately, stopping such use may have little or no impact on farm profits and food costs. And recent years have seen many such uses discouraged or prohibited in several countries.

Farms need sufficient support and remuneration to transition to better systems—as a matter of urgency. The public can help support good farming practices, and avoid pressurizing veterinary and anthropic medics for drugs they do not need, and always finish the prescribed course of antibiotics. It is a revealing fact that the use—and perhaps misuse—of antibiotics seems to vary between countries. The EU has banned using most antibiotics to promote growth in farm animals, but this practice is often common in many other countries. Within Europe, Denmark and Sweden have strict policies on using drugs for humans and animals, and they have low levels of resistance. Italy has appeared to be less discriminating and has increasing levels of resistance.

In some countries such as Greece and China, people may actually be able to buy anti-microbials over the counter.

There is some debate as to whether, and to what extent, resistant microbes spread from non-human animals to humans. There is certainly the *potential* for resistance to spread, and animal care and meat processing should minimize this potential. However, this is not the same as evidence that drug use in animals is causing resistance. In the UK, human medical use of antibiotics is 2.4 times greater than it is in veterinary use (per kg of patient). Plus, in the vast majority of cases (from studies in Denmark, Germany, the Netherlands, Sweden, and the UK), the resistant bacteria found in humans appear genetically different to those found in other species. Our efforts to prevent the development of resistant microbes need to focus on where those microbes are developed and spread.

Comparative medicine

Veterinary research can help us to a better general understanding of diseases' causes and mechanisms, reliable clinical signs and tests, and safe, effective treatments. Scientists dissect (when dead), vivisect (while alive), or experiment upon animals in order to understand their biology and pathology. Scientists also cause illnesses and injuries in non-human animals in a laboratory through genetic manipulation, toxic doses of chemicals, and surgery (e.g. to close blood vessels) in order to understand diseases occurring outside of the laboratory. They may also test drugs on laboratory animals before using them on patients. Such studies can be intended to help human or non-human patients.

Laboratory research and tests have potential advantages. Small numbers of animals can be used under controlled conditions, allowing scientists to really focus on particular detailed research questions before applying the findings to larger numbers of patients. Tissue samples and cells may be used (i.e. not making animals feel ill). Laboratory species such as mice, rats, and fish are quick to breed and relatively cheap to keep in laboratory conditions. But laboratory animal research also has its disadvantages. Animals are deliberately genetically modified, bred, or sometimes captured from the wild; kept captive; and made unwell. The development of treatments may be delayed while laboratory tests are conducted, and some patients may suffer or die in the meantime. And animals may suffer in laboratory environments that do not meet their needs. Such stress can make the data less valuable, quite apart from ethical considerations of this treatment. In many countries, laws try to reduce these harms but they have not been eliminated.

Another concern is that laboratory research does not study 'real-life' diseases in naturally occurring patients. While the majority of laboratory animals are mice, rats, and fish, most real patients are humans, farm animals, dogs, and horses. Many laboratory animals live in unnatural (and potentially stressful) conditions and their illnesses are man-made: a genetically modified, surgically altered rat living in a lab is fortunately not much like many human patients. For example, cancers that occur spontaneously in humans are deliberately created in laboratory mice through artificial means (e.g. by adding new genes or grafting human cancer tissues onto them, and then giving drugs to stop their immune system rejecting the transplant). Many of these models are really only used because they are traditional—or in scientists' terms, they are 'well-established models'.

In comparison, real-life patients' cancers have very complex underlying genetic and environmental causes. They may also react very differently from induced tumours in laboratory rodents. They may occur in different tissues, respond to drugs in different ways, and spread or recur differently. Patients are complex individuals living in a multi-dimensional world. As a result, such studies may give misleading information. Misleading information may lead to a risk that we dismiss valuable treatments because they have not worked in laboratories; or that we develop drugs because they do work in labs but which later prove to be dangerous for our patients. Most animal studies do not directly lead to treatments that are used for patients. We should be aiming to end the use of live animals in harmful research, veterinary or otherwise.

Perhaps part of the problem is the aim of the research. There is a danger of biomedical science seeing animals only as tools to study biological mechanisms, just in order to extrapolate the findings for human patients. Such research inherently damages the health of the animal as an individual, and misses the empathy and ethics you would hope to find in anthropic medical practice. This risks a prismatic and biased appreciation of those animals and their biology that is very different from the understanding clinicians want to gain for their patients. Wherever possible, studies should avoid affecting the physical or mental health of suffering animals. But where studies *do* use live animals, scientists should consider them not as tools or biological models, but as whole, live, sentient, individual patients.

Outside the laboratory

Given the ethical concerns around animal experimentation, there is some excitement about the current opportunities to learn from animals without deliberately making them ill or keeping them in laboratories. Rather than trying to create unnatural diseases in laboratory conditions, it seems better to learn from actually treating real-life diseases in veterinary patients who are already ill. Such research can include the study of diseases, their causes, and the effects of drugs using data from veterinary clinical trials, diagnostics, or epidemiological studies. This can help to develop new treatments for all species.

For example, much of the seminal work on in-vitro fertilization was done by veterinary scientists treating sheep. Another example is that veterinarians have long used magnets to capture metal in the stomachs of cows, who sometimes swallow wires hidden in silage.

More recently, medical scientists have developed a magnetic mini-robot to capture metal in the stomachs of humans, who sometimes swallow objects like batteries. There are differences in how these treatments are used—in particular, the cow magnet usually stays in her stomach permanently (to find out if a cow has a magnet in her stomach, you can place a compass near her chest), whereas the human robot will be removed once it has done its job—but the basic idea is one that has moved from cows to humans.

Another area of particular interest is dog cancer and genetic diseases, particularly given the prominence of cancer in pet dogs and our understanding of their genetics. Treating their cancers can help us learn about how cancers work in all species. For example, scientists have recently trialled ways to get enough anti-cancer drugs into dog organs, which have helped develop similar treatments for humans. Nanoparticles (made from bits of bacteria) can carry drugs into the brain where they can kill human or dog tumour cells. Both human and pet dog lymphoma cells might be killed by a strain of the Newcastle disease virus. Other cancers might be killed by distemper or measles viruses.

Research on cancers in pet dogs may provide much better data than laboratory experiments. Dogs, and their cancers, are generally more similar to humans than the mice cancers that scientists create. Spontaneous cancers in pet dogs and humans are often similar in their clinical presentation, cellular features, molecules, response to therapy, and drug resistance. Many occur in similar places (e.g. some bone cancers and non-Hodgkin's lymphoma). Dogs and humans also share human environments, live until old age, and are given extensive medical treatment, and so they may be exposed to similar risk factors and causes. Cancers in real-world animal populations also have a degree of variation that is similar to the variation found in human cancers, due to differences in patients' genetics, anatomy, physiology, lifestyle, concurrent diseases, experience of illness, and response to the disease.

Studying real-world dog cancers can also help us understand the genetic bases for cancers. Dogs and humans also share many genes (which mice do not), and dog and human cancers may have similar genetic bases (e.g. several colon, rectal, bone, and soft tissue tumours). Indeed, the risks of certain cancers in particular dog breeds can be linked to their breeds, family tree, and now-mapped genome. Such data may be even more useful than human data, given that dogs have larger litter sizes and shorter generation gaps (making family studies easier), simpler genetics (due to the genetic bottleneck that occurred during domestication), an often higher degree of inbreeding (amongst some pedigrees), and several genetic separations between populations (as people want 'pure' breeds). Recent advances are also making dog gene-sequencing technologies increasingly faster and cheaper in practice.

Getting data from such veterinary treatments seems generally preferable to using animals in laboratory studies. Reducing the reliance on laboratory testing may mean that drugs can get to human and animal patients sooner—so that patients may avoid having delayed treatment—and that drugs are not wrongly discounted because they did not work in laboratories or humans. Using real-life patients avoids the need to create diseased animals in laboratory studies. (The ethical questions about creating unhealthy pedigrees are a separate issue—while such problems exist, it seems sensible to use the data obtained from treating them.) It becomes morally harder to justify creating ill animals when there are already ill animals you could help, and thereby get good or better data at the same time.

Such veterinary trials should also have an empathetic attitude that is more compatible with the ultimate aim of helping patients. In human and veterinary medicine, clinicians need to resolve ethical questions about when it is acceptable to use an 'experimental' drug on a patient (human or non-human), and carefully ensure that all treatments are beneficial to those patients—as all medics should. In fact, applying ethical standards to trials involving patients of non-human species may mean treatments and trials are designed to be more similar to those that would be applied to humans. There will remain differences, such as those regarding euthanasia and consent, but the basic respectful principles should be the same. Using data from studies in dogs may also have added benefits such as bringing veterinary and anthropic medicine closer together (e.g. into mainstream medical cancer journals).

Healthy relations

Another link between human and non-human animal health is in our relationships with each other. There is increasing evidence that the companionship of healthy pets can confer a range of health benefits (although the evidence for some links may be over-stated). Pet owning appears to improve humans' cardiovascular function, their loyal companionship can help people cope with acute stress, and dog walking can encourage owners to exercise and to meet other dog walkers socially. Such links provide opportunities for doctors and veterinarians to work together to improve the health of both their patients given that many owners *and* many animals are overweight or even obese, or are socially isolated from their own species. The future development of mobile technologies and lifestyle applications will doubtless lead to further entrepreneurial efforts to link ways to improve owner and pet health.

There also appear to be advantages for human children and young animals growing up together, particularly in promoting good mental health. Children in homes with pets may have higher self-esteem, better social skills, and more interactive families. Puppies and kittens in homes with children can get used to them, finding them less scary when they get older. And, of course, children and pets can form enormously beneficial bonds, such as that between Owen Howkins, a boy with Schwartz-Jampel Syndrome, which causes painful, chronic muscle contractions, and Haatchi, his three-legged Anatolian shepherd dog who lost

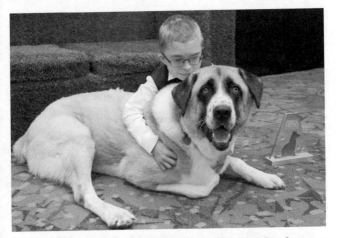

12. **Owen and Haatchi's is a wonderful story of how their love has helped them cope with their medical conditions together.**

his leg and tail when he was hit by a train after being tied to a railway line. Haatchi has helped Owen cope in his difficulties, take his medicine, and go through painful physiotherapy (Figure 12), while Haatchi has benefited from companionship with Owen in his own physically diminished state.

There are, sadly, also downsides to human relationships with other animals (Figure 13). Some people may mistreat both vulnerable non-human animals and vulnerable children or other dependants. Injuries to both can include cigarette burns, fractures from victims being swung, or genital damage. Many patients may be seen with multiple or repeated injuries. Some patients become fearful towards to their guardian, sometimes showing a 'frozen watchfulness', but others may still appear very loving to their abuser (in humans this is sometimes described as Stockholm syndrome). While the research on animal abuse tends to focus on dogs, one study in Brazil actually found that cats were more commonly victimized. Of course, many victims of abuse will not

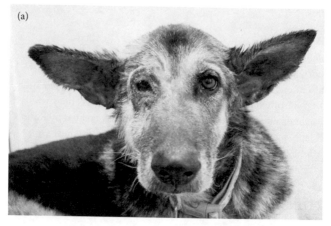

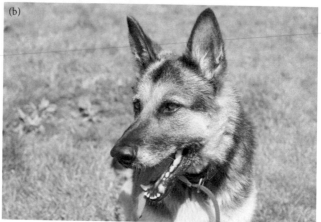

13. This dog was the victim of neglect that had caused significant suffering (a); but recovered after veterinary attention and good care (b).

be taken to receive medical care and, for both doctors and veterinarians, abuse can be hard to spot in the first place.

A prominent theory is that the underlying personality or mental health issues in the abuser can prompt them to mistreat both humans and other animals.

A specific form of abuse seen in children and animals is where a guardian takes their child or pet for medical attention, either when they are not actually ill or for illnesses that have been deliberately caused by that carer. Guardians may present their pets or children for medical care in order to gain sympathy or attention. This is known as Munchausen syndrome, named after Baron Munchausen, a fictional 18th-century mercenary who became addicted to lying about his adventures, created by Rudolf Raspe (and loosely based on a real baron called Freiherr von Münchhausen) in his 1785 book, *Baron Munchausen's Narrative of his Marvellous Travels and Campaigns in Russia* (the character has also appeared in many films, including the 1988 Terry Gilliam film, *The Adventures of Baron Munchausen*). These patients may end up receiving unnecessary, unpleasant, or even risky medical attention. Some guardians may even give their victims a variety of drugs or poisons in order to create signs of illness in the first place. There has been some valuable work on the mental health of such guardians, although that research is in the early stages in terms of being identified in animal abuse.

We all stand together

The link between human and non-human animal health has been present from the start of modern medicine. Pioneers such as Giovanni Lancisi, Rudolf Virchow (who coined the term 'zoonosis' to mean diseases that cross species to humans), and William Osler argued that there should be no dividing lines within an overall concept of medicine. The last two decades have seen some attempts to re-forge this link. A lot of effort has gone into trying to sketch out an over-arching concept of what is, essentially, a simple idea: the health of human and non-human animals is linked (and linked also, as discussed in Chapter 6, within the overall health of the environment that we all inhabit). What is important is that experts work together, transcending each specialism, and *all* focus our concern on the health of *all* animals.

There is a real danger in considering animal health to be important only insofar as it affects humans' physical health. Diseases like avian influenza have helped motivate collaboration, and the response to epidemics of this influenza is sometimes cited as representing a success story in building a new collaborative approach. But it is difficult to say that this was a success in terms of improving animal health, given that the main treatment for the problem was widespread poultry culling. To really make a difference for human and non-human health, it would be better to prevent the development and spread of new viral strains in all species by carefully examining how farm chickens, pigs, and other animals are reared. Similarly, we should not need definitive evidence linking SARS and civets to stop the harmful practices associated with civet farming and its use in coffee production—where coffee beans eaten and defecated by caged civets are sold as a premium product.

Human society needs to consider human and non-human animal health together. We can consider how the diets of farmed animals affect both their health and the health of the people and other animals who eat their produce. We can consider the lifestyle causes and effects of cancer in both humans and their pets. Globally, we can coordinate health agencies, such as the WHO and the OIE. Locally, we can collaborate as veterinary and anthropic medical practices, for example by organizing dog walking or local education groups. And we should consider animal health not just as a list of microbes that can infect humans, but as a range of physical, mental, and social aspects that affect a range of animals, especially as we gain increasing scientific understanding of how human and non-human animals have similar needs and can suffer in similar ways.

Indeed, we might think of all animals—human and non-human—as part of the same 'herd'. Members of this herd share a wide range of genes, biological characteristics, and environmental conditions. The members of this herd interact socially, often enjoying (or fearing) each other's company, and help one another to cope with challenges. These interactions mean problems can spread between members of that herd, depending on how they live and how they interact. Different individuals may be affected in different ways, depending on how well they can resist or cope with diseases, which, in turn, depends on how well cared for they are. Alternatively, we can think of humans and other animals as being part of an interconnected ecosystem, where any problems for one species can have serious knock-on effects. This herd, or ecosystem, is becoming increasingly global, as we shall discuss in Chapter 6.

To work together, we need to overcome distinctions that hinder comparisons between species. We sometimes consider human and animal health-related quality of life very differently. We avoid applying words like 'symptoms' to animals. We may forget or be disproportionately sceptical that animals feel bad when they are ill, hurt, or mistreated. We subject other vertebrate animals to illnesses or environmental conditions that we would consider unacceptable in humans. We use animals in experiments that bear little resemblance to the real-life situations of the patients we want to help. Indeed, we use the term 'medical' as if it applies only to humans, rather than recognizing that there are multiple specialisms within 'medicine'. These differences are cultural, social, and ethical rather than scientific, but that may actually make them easier to overcome if we can be reflective, honourable, and open-minded enough.

Chapter 6
Global veterinary medicine

The global herd

We live in a global society. And this is just as much the case
for veterinary medicine as it is for our food industry and our
climate. The cells, microbes, parasites, and genes that cause
disease may be tiny, but they can travel large distances around the
planet. In other words, geography is no longer a major barrier to
the transmission of either germs or genes, or the interaction of
different animals. Consequently, many of the key issues affecting
ourselves, our animals, and our environments involve not just
isolated individuals or populations but also the increasingly
inter-connected continents. We now need to think of all
animals worldwide as a single population—herd medicine
on a global scale.

Animals themselves have been spread around the world, moving
away from their original habitats. Chickens, descended from
a species native to Asia, are today farmed extensively in the
Americas. Turkeys, which were wild in North America, are now
raised in Asia. Guinea pigs, which are originally from the Andes,
are farmed in Africa. Reptiles and birds are kept as pets far from
their original countries—bearded dragons and budgerigars are
originally Australian; parrots are African or South American;
golden hamsters are Syrian; and chinchillas originally come from

Chile, Peru, Argentina, and Bolivia (although they are now extinct or endangered in those countries). Humans have spread abroad wild animals such as deer, camels, pigs, foxes, mink, cats, rats, rabbits, wallabies, pigeons, parakeets, pheasants, finches, geese, geckos, snakes, terrapins, toads, trout, carp, and crabs. Islands like New Zealand have a litany of introduced species, including cows (for farming) and Australian brushtail possums (for fur).

In farming, the worldwide use of a small number of common animal species and breeds may have particularly increased the risks and impacts of global disease. If a microbe infects pigs or chickens (or humans), it can now find hosts worldwide. Indeed, many farm animals have been bred so that they are even more similar to each other: a few strains of chickens from genetically related breeding stock are used across the world. These animals tend to share similar genes, similar immune systems, and similar disease susceptibilities, and are usually kept in similar conditions. If those strains are susceptible to a particular microbe or genetic problem, the resulting disease could spread through the international 'herd' and potentially wipe out large proportions of that global population.

The international distribution of animals and animal products can also lead to the spread of their microbes and genes. This can spread diseases, particularly when the animals are moved faster than their diseases' incubation periods. Rift Valley fever was probably spread to the Arabian peninsula in cattle from Africa. Humans took tuberculosis into New Zealand, probably in imported cows (or perhaps imported deer or the humans themselves). The imported possums then got infected—and are now being killed in an attempt to reduce the risk of tuberculosis in cows. Humans also spread the invertebrates that transmit microbes, such as insects and ticks, outside of their own native habitats. Migrating or holidaying humans can carry animal microbes on or in our bodies and possessions. The international spread of microbes can also cause a mixing of different microbes that otherwise would never have met, potentially leading to them sharing drug resistance or developing into new strains.

Sometimes, the international spread of microbes brings them into contact with naive populations. A classic example is the pox virus spread by grey squirrels, imported from North America, to red squirrels in the UK. (The grey squirrels also out-compete reds for resources—but often the red squirrels have already been killed by the disease spreading from the grey squirrels' arrival in an area). Grey squirrels have such a high degree of immunity that they can spread the virus with little or no effect on themselves, whereas red squirrels are naive to the virus with nearly all victims dying—and usually very quickly. The situation bears a horrid resemblance to the contrary spread of European smallpox in the Americas—which killed off almost all of the indigenous human populations (although smallpox also killed many of the immigrant populations too). Of course, it's not the greys' fault.

Another example is the chytrid fungus that has devastated wild amphibians across the world, most recently in Southeast Asia. The fungus was probably recently spread from Africa by human trade in African clawed toads and perhaps also in captive American bullfrogs. Like many diseases, it was probably not that damaging to the African animals (because otherwise it would likely have already wiped out the populations on which its lifecycle depends). But once it spread to naive animals abroad, who lack effective immunity, it has been devastating for wild amphibians across the world. Sadly, a second, related species of fungus has recently been found that affects salamanders.

Of course, the spread of infectious diseases is not completely new. Historic bubonic plagues probably started in Mongolian marmots before being spread by fleas on rats. Migrating animals have been connecting continents for millennia, potentially spreading diseases (nowadays including birds carrying avian influenza and ticks carrying *Borrelia*). West Nile virus often seems to travel along bird migratory routes, devastating local bird populations—although the initial introduction of the virus into the USA was probably due to humans transporting infected animals or mosquitoes. (Amazingly, some northern wheatear birds were recently found to travel from Africa to North America, but there is no evidence they are responsible for spreading disease.) What is new is the sheer scale of our international connections that allow a greater scale of disease spread.

One promising way to better understand the spread of disease across continents is by considering the health of the global population of animals as one global herd or ecosystem. Veterinarians are skilled in understanding how diseases spread on a farm, in a breed, or in a single land-mass. Some of the underlying veterinary scientific principles can help us understand disease worldwide—so long as they are appropriately adapted. Such a 'global herd' approach may help us find better ways to prevent the spread of diseases and minimize their impacts. This should inspire veterinary and anthropic medical scientists in every country to give more attention to the health of animals in other countries who might be future sources of infection to their own. This means supporting veterinary science in countries where it is less developed.

Coping with what lies ahead

Veterinary science will increasingly need to treat the effects of human activity on animals' environments, both locally and globally. Our activities can damage animals' health directly or mean their natural biology and behaviour no longer fit their altered or man-made environments. Animals may need treatment after contamination by oil spills, road accident injuries, starvation, or habitat destruction (Figure 14). Others may need medical help after becoming entangled in traps or man-made debris. These include animals caught in snares; waterbirds who swallow discarded fishing lines; turtles who eat plastic bags after

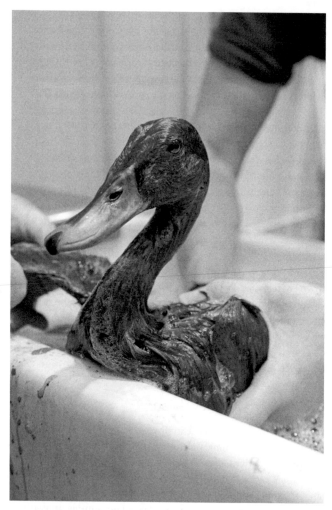

14. Decontamination of a bird covered in oil.

mistaking them for jellyfish; marine animals caught in 'ghost nets' that fishermen have either lost or deliberately discarded; pigeons whose toes get encircled by discarded string or fishing line; and seabirds who make nests from plastic debris as if it were a natural, biodegradable material. Veterinarians may treat a few of these animals, but attention is better paid to prevention.

Veterinarians can also try to minimize the damage caused by humans taking animals from the wild. These animals are taken from their natural environment and sometimes this means also from their familiar family or social groups. They may be transported long distances into new, man-made environments to be kept in zoological exhibits, circuses, aquaria, vivariums, cages, human homes, or fields in very different climates. The stress of this displacement can bring out diseases with which they were otherwise coping or it can lead to mental health disorders, which we sometimes see expressed in the repetitive behaviours of some captive, previously wild animals. They may carry microbes or parasites with them, or encounter new ones in their new environments. Their removal from a social group may cause loss and disruption to the animals left behind, unbalancing natural ecosystems, reducing biodiversity, and endangering their own species. Veterinarians can sometimes help the individual animals to cope with the effects of their displacement, but it is harder to repair an ecosystem.

Other effects of human activity may lead to veterinary health problems by affecting animal numbers and movements. Habitat destruction through the building of new roads, for example, or other disruptions that cause the loss of a species' predators or prey may negatively impact on animal groups, making them more infectious, vulnerable, stressed, or inbred. For example, in the northern USA, ongoing disruption by human de-forestation and re-forestation has disturbed wildlife and fragmented their habitats, driving the spread of *Borrelia* infections. In more tropical regions, the spread of microbes like *Leishmania* and

Trypanosomes has been linked to land use changes such as logging and mining. One study found that red colobus monkeys had more worms where more de-forestation had occurred, perhaps because they came into contact with humans. More generally, human activity often brings animals into close contact with humans or domestic animals. For example, foxes and bobcats near urban environments may come into contact with microbes and parasites from dogs and cats.

With global warming, increased local temperatures may also cause more cases of hyperthermia, and the heat may reduce animals' immunity, fertility, and productivity (in 2011, heat waves cost farmers over US$1 billion). Droughts may cause dehydration (particularly in animals producing milk), and can worsen pasture quality or crops that are used to feed animals. Floods can spread diseases such as Leptospirosis and Rift Valley fever. Many of these health problems have been traditionally found in developing countries, and so they have attracted limited investment in research. But worldwide, veterinary science will increasingly need to adapt in order to be able to provide treatment for such conditions.

In particular, veterinarians may see several serious diseases increasing their range, as our climate changes and areas become warmer (or colder) and wetter (or drier) in ways that favour the spread of microbes or the animals that can carry them. Many economically important or dangerous diseases usually found in warm areas appear to be expanding to new areas, such as *Leishmania*, Rift Valley fever, and West Nile diseases. The spread of Nipah was probably partly down to climatic changes (alongside the methods used to raise pigs). In Tunisia, global warming may increase the range of desert plants eaten by sand rats who may spread *Leishmania*. Local land-use changes such as man-made lakes may also provide environments for parasite hosts or breeding grounds for insects that can carry disease.

Some forms of pollution, such as oil spills, are obvious. Veterinary science can identify how best to treat such disasters (and if in some instances euthanasia is best for the animals involved). However, many of the effects of pollution are subtler and wider. The long-term exposure to pollutants may—for human and non-human animals—lead to the risk of health problems (e.g. respiratory disease or cancer from air pollution or cigarette smoke). Animals' bodies may be unable to detoxify or excrete unnatural chemicals, which can build up to high levels. Consequently, some animals may be at particular risk, such as fish poisoned by heavy metals or agricultural pesticides that leak into the water; or predatory fish who eat any contaminated smaller fish. Fish veterinarians may even need to treat diseases related to pollution or poor water quality due to fertilizers causing algae to grow and use up the oxygen needed by the microbes that would otherwise keep the water clean. Some of these problems may be caused by veterinarians: for example the widespread use of the anti-inflammatory diclofenac for farm animals, which is highly toxic to vultures and almost wiped out several species in the Indian subcontinent.

Humans may also build habitats for humans and domestic animals closer to those of wild animals, increasing their exposure to each other and to any refuse. Microbes such as influenza and Nipah viruses may then 'spill over' from humans or domestic animals to wild animals living nearby, or vice-versa. Of particular concern is cross-contamination between humans, poultry, and wild birds. Where large numbers of poultry are kept together, microbes can build up and potentially mutate before infecting a wild animal or human. Alternatively, infection from a wild animal or human can spread through flocks quickly and disastrously, going on to infect further wild animals, any humans who work there, or any animals who eat infected meat or eggs. These 'plagues' can be difficult to control—hence measures often involve widespread culling.

As urban environments expand (and natural environments shrink), some wildlife also make use of human habitats, slums, and rubbish dumps. These animals may be susceptible to microbes found in humans or other urban animals. Furthermore, even if urban animals seem remarkably adaptive, their fit in the urban environment is still catching up in evolutionary terms. So animals (including humans) in urban environments may cope less well and be generally less healthy. They may also be found at greater population densities than in the wild (again, including humans), increasing the potential spread. Veterinarians need to treat infected animals and to manage the risks to humans and other animals. Recent years have begun to see a more collaborative approach between human, veterinary, and environmental sciences, and rabies can be cost-effectively controlled by vaccinating stray dogs and wildlife (perhaps more effectively even than just vaccinating the human population).

As humans change the global and local environments, veterinary science needs to get better at predicting and preventing the emergence and spread of diseases and, when some still do inevitably occur, to identify them and respond to them quickly, effectively, and proportionately. However, it is not always possible to accurately predict how our activities will impact on particular habitats, and affect animal health within and outside that habitat. Ecosystems represent complex interconnections between animals and their environment, and altering one aspect of them can have unpredictable effects. Probably the best strategy—for prevention—is to leave the remaining natural environments alone.

Veterinary conservation

As human activities impact on wild animals, this can lead to reductions in biodiversity and threaten the existence of particular species. Improving wildlife health is a key part of conservation, to offset the effects of natural processes and human activity. Veterinary science has a clear role in the conservation of species

and biodiversity by helping protect healthy animals and treat
ill animals.

Most obviously, veterinarians can treat individual endangered
animals, which can help maintain populations when numbers are
so critically low that the survival of individual animals makes all
the difference. For example, the Northern white rhinoceros has
only one male and two females left alive (one other having died
while this book was being written), so the survival of the species
depends entirely on the continued health of those individual
animals. Sadly, it is almost certainly already too late for other
rhinoceroses, such as the Western black rhinoceros, who have
already been declared extinct. Releasing rehabilitated animals
can also mean those animals continue to have their beneficial
impact on their ecosystem, eating or being eaten, competing
with other animals, spreading seeds, and fertilizing soils. The
treatment of key animals may stop their ecosystem 'unravelling'
because all animals in an environment are interlinked.

However, just as for individual animals, prevention is better
than cure. The aim should not be simply to patch up ill animals,
but also to stop them becoming injured or ill in the first place.
Veterinary scientific methods can help work out why animals
get ill or injured, and reduce those causes. Veterinarians can
help control the spread of diseases such as retroviruses and
Chlamydia in koalas, and ranavirus and chytrid fungus in
amphibians. They can vaccinate wild animals (e.g. against rabies).
They can try to improve the genetics of wild populations,
particularly in groups made small (e.g. due to poaching) or
isolated (e.g. due to habitat destruction), by reducing inbreeding
and selecting good combinations of mates, and by tracking
animals' choices of mates by examining their DNA.

By the same logic, veterinary science can help us avoid human
activities that spread diseases through wild populations. It can help
us see where habitat destruction might cause animals to move

away; where farmed animals might pose a risk to (as well as from) local wildlife; and where capturing animals for pets can spread disease. A number of the diseases in this book have involved human activity spreading the microbes that have devastated local populations. The spread of diseases among the global herd of domestic animals can easily 'spill over' into the wild populations—microbes can cross both ways. More generally, habitat damage and climate changes may make animals less able to cope with diseases, and thus become more vulnerable to significant effects.

Veterinary science can consider conservation using the concepts that apply to 'herds'. Veterinarians are used to considering the overall health of populations of animals, and balancing the interests of different individuals within a species or across multiple species. Veterinary science can consider how the health of one animal may impact on others, and how to obtain the best health overall. Veterinary concepts and approaches can be applied to an individual, and then to a herd, to an ecosystem, and even to the whole world—of humans, non-human animals, and other species. Just like a body is made up of cells and organs, interacting in ways that are far more complex than the sum of its parts, so an ecosystem is an interaction of all its members. Our effects on one part can have unpredictable impacts on other parts, or the ecosystem as a whole.

Our veterinary preventive aims make it important to be concerned about all animals and the whole ecosystem. Veterinary science may most easily be applied to large mammal species, who are often the most 'charismatic' animals in each ecosystem (or in zoological collections) and directly affected by prominent unethical human activities (e.g. big game hunting). But the inter-linkages between species mean protecting the health of natural ecologies requires concern about the health of all animals: mammals, birds, reptiles, fish, amphibians, insects, corals, etc. (and plants, fungi, and many microbes) who help maintain the system's balance. Our 'herd' is the entire global ecosystem.

Careful conservation

Veterinary science can also help to ensure that our wildlife management efforts minimize the possible harms to animal health. Just as clinicians try to avoid side-effects when treating individual patients, society should also try to avoid the unintended, negative consequences of trying to improve our environment's health.

Veterinary science can help us avoid unintended consequences when trying to save or breed endangered animals. The good intention of saving a species should not mean that individual animals are then kept alive at any cost—especially when this merely offsets or delays problems caused by ongoing human activities. Conservationists need to evaluate the suffering caused by confinement (e.g. during breeding programmes), extending lifespans (e.g. to save the last member of a species), or veterinary treatment (e.g. after poacher injuries), recognizing that wild animals may suffer from being restrained in captivity and find human contact extremely distressing.

Similarly, veterinary science can help avoid spreading disease when animals are moved, for example to save them from habitat destruction in their native geographies. Relocating animals can spread diseases that may be very damaging to any new neighbours who lack their immunity. Veterinary science can select healthier animals to be moved, and put adequate quarantine and biosecurity measures in place. By understanding the microbes and the animals, veterinary science can help work out how microbes or parasites might survive in the environment and affect local populations (e.g. whether they have the hosts for parasites' earlier life stages).

At the same time, veterinary science can help give the moved animals a better chance at survival. Being moved can place animals in unfamiliar environments, with unfamiliar competition and unfamiliar microbes. Indeed, one might expect relocated animals to meet more new diseases than they bring. There is little benefit (and much harm) in treating and curing animals only for them to starve or die more slowly. A scientific understanding of the genetics of the local and relocated animals can also help assess where best to move the animals to ensure their best possible genetic health.

Veterinary science can help us improve how—and whether—to limit wild populations, such as by killing animals or by introducing predators or diseases like myxomatosis. Veterinary science can help identify where these might make animals suffer directly or have knock-on effects on the health of the ecosystem, other animals, or humans. In Africa, killing leopards can increase baboon populations, which might then spread parasites to humans. In the savannah, destroying the habitats of insects that spread diseases like sleeping sickness may have wider effects on local ecosystems. In England, autopsies suggested many of the badgers killed to tackle tuberculosis appeared to have suffered significantly because the shots missed the target area. Sometimes veterinary science shows it is better not to attempt to control wild populations.

By considering the health of all the animals and ecosystems worldwide, as one population, environmental impacts can be recognized not only as problems in themselves, but also as clinical signs of underlying problems. In an individual animal, weight loss may be a sign of an underlying disease. In a species, population decreases may also be a sign of an underlying, life-threatening problem. This way of thinking can help guide our decisions on what to do. In individual animals, veterinarians should not only treat the symptoms of a problem, but try to tackle the root causes. So too, in the 'world herd', the focus should be less on saving the last of a doomed species (especially if doing so goes against the interests of those individual animals) and more on dealing with the causes of biodiversity loss: habitat destruction, climate change, pollution, etc.

Future farming

Perhaps the most exciting promise of veterinary science is how it can help farmers avoid some of the physical and mental health problems that particular farming systems can cause in their animal stocks, and thereby make the systems more sustainable and profitable for farmers. Gradually, veterinary science is eliminating infectious diseases such as bovine tuberculosis, foot and mouth, some strains of scrapie, and goat plague (albeit while new ones are being discovered). Veterinary science can re-design farming systems to reduce the need for antibiotics and preventive surgery; it can help breed animals who can cope better in farming systems, while avoiding creating new genetic problems.

It is important such progress avoids creating a situation where animals are being constantly adapted to fit new, badly designed farming systems that place additional pressure on them. Instead, veterinary science can help ensure farming methods fit the animals as they are. It is also important that developing industries do not misguidedly adopt as 'new' the outdated systems that other industries are moving away from. Developing countries have the chance to catch up (and overtake) by avoiding methods that have been used in the developed world that place large numbers of animals in impoverished and stressful situations, with all the accompanying health and ethical concerns they entail.

The pressures that our farming styles place on animals are ultimately due to pressure placed on farmers themselves by retailers and ultimately from us, the consumers. So, to achieve healthy farming, good farmers need to be supported financially, partly by avoiding excessive competition that requires cutting costs at the expense of the animal, the farmers, or the environment. Farm subsidies, trade agreements, and other market incentives need to include animal, human, and environmental health as core values. The financial bottom line should be balanced with the other objectives of protecting farmers, customers, public safety, the environment, and animals themselves. For example, given the increasing importance of fish farming, veterinary science has a vital role in ensuring the farmed products of crustacea, shellfish, and finfish are safe, healthy, nutritious, and produced in ways that minimize any impact on the local and global environment.

Indeed, greater input from veterinary science can help with global economic efforts. Healthier animals can improve financial security for farmers and food security for consumers. Healthier animals should survive longer, produce more, grow faster, and need fewer medicines. Indeed, recent evidence suggests routinely using antibiotics to avoid low-grade disease may actually cost farms more than it saves. Farmers with healthier animals may also be able to charge consumers more, or perhaps receive subsidies from forward-thinking governments. Supporting subsistence and small-scale farming may also help to slow the increase in poverty, given estimates that roughly two-thirds of the world's poor depend on livestock. Farmers may then have the money to invest in giving their animals good food, rest, veterinary care, tack, and housing. Reduced poverty may also reduce practices that increase the risk of diseases spreading across species, such as eating bushmeat or providing livestock with unhygienic living conditions.

Preventing diseases can cost more in the short-term but save money in the long-term. Poor tack and care for working animals can make them less able to make money for their owners. Trying to eradicate outbreaks of avian influenza has cost billions of dollars. Tackling Nipah almost destroyed the Malaysian pig industry, which was worth many billions of dollars. The SARS outbreak led to serious losses to tourism industries and financial markets. Often these costs are not borne by the people (or countries) whose poor practices have actually caused the disease outbreaks in the first place, and many countries can ill afford the health costs of human diseases that have come from farm (or wild) animals. So governments may need to ensure that responsibilities are placed where they should be. Often, better care leads to more profit—or, at least, financial sustainability—the limiting factor for the farmers is having the cash-flow needed to invest in future returns.

Improving food security is arguably not about maximizing production in developed countries that have problems of obesity and excessive pollution. It is estimated that up to 70 per cent of the global human food intake is provided by pastoral and smallholder farms (Figure 15). So development efforts need to be aimed at supporting smallholder farmers in developing countries to maximize their outputs. This is not just about giving them animals. Organizations who are involved in placing livestock in some of their projects should ensure that they are productive, otherwise such efforts are effectively burdening otherwise very poor people with very large pets. It is also important to ensure that the welfare of those animals will be maintained, so they are not simply being sent to suffer.

Veterinary science may help protect the global environment. Some farming leads to the production of large amounts of methane—not counting the gases released in the practice of de-forestation to make space. For many years, veterinary scientists have been looking for ways to reduce the amount of methane produced by cow, sheep, and goat digestion. Some attempt to change their diet (e.g. altering the amounts of tannins in feeds), the microbes in their stomachs, or their genetics (e.g. selecting sheep or cows who emit less methane). Unfortunately, several promising methods seem to risk creating an increase in health problems such as rumen acidosis, toxicity, liver abscesses, or decreased feed efficiency. In fact, using healthy, long-living, grass-fed cows might reduce methane production by 15–30 per cent, as well as helping the cows and farmers through lower infertility, lameness, udder infections, and heat stress. Other research suggests methane is not as bad for the environment as previously thought.

We need to consider an approach that incorporates the health and well-being of animals, farmers, consumers, local environments, and the global herd and ecosystem. By doing so, we can achieve all of the aims contained in veterinary oaths. Certain farming systems require fewer resources; provide better lives for the animals and farmers in terms of environments, economics, and fairness; ensure animals are resilient to potential challenges; provide more nutritious and safer meat, eggs, and milk; and avoid excessive pollution. Veterinary scientists can combine helping individual animals and farms with challenging poor farming practices, as we understand more about the potential longer term costs in terms of animal welfare, obesity, pollution, antibiotic resistance, and reduced biodiversity.

Epilogue: the future of veterinary medicine

Veterinary science stands on the edge of a bright new future. It is essential to the health, growth, function, resilience, and well-being of individual patients, herds, ecosystems, economies, societies, and environments—across species and across the world. It can repair damage done by diseases and human activity. It can tackle old and new diseases as they cause problems, and prevent some problems from even happening. It can scientifically inform fundamental changes in how we interact with animals, and new generations of veterinary scientists can push for changes within our professional lifetimes.

A primary veterinary aim is to help non-human animals, who can get ill and suffer just as humans can. But veterinary science is essential to protecting the health of humans, economies, and the environment. It serves the inter-connected herd and global ecosystem that includes our farming, trade, travel, and wildlife. We need to think scientifically about the unpredictable disease risks of having millions of genetically similar, stressed, immunologically naive animals kept in densely populated conditions for many generations—and then shipped around the world in order for them to be eaten by other animals. We know that compassionate care for those animals can be key to protecting everyone's welfare and preventing catastrophic diseases. We know we need adequate veterinary infrastructures in all countries—in public, private, and charity sectors—to protect humans and non-humans alike.

Rather than the care of animals being seen as a luxury only possible in the developed world, it should be seen as an integral part of helping humans, animals, and the environment worldwide. We fear various global problems—if not crises—including environmental pollution, climate change, species eradication, and altered human lifestyles. Veterinary science can help tackle—or avert—these problems through its approach to hard facts; to positioning and prioritizing problems; and to pragmatic problem-solving. Increasingly the scientific matters will need to be seen within their political, societal, and historical contexts.

This widens the philosophy of veterinary science to encompass global concerns for economic stability, food security, and social justice. Our economic concerns should focus on what is really valuable—for everyone. Our concern to stop poverty should prevent behaviours such as de-forestation, pollution, and over-consumption. Our concern for food security should focus on healthy, resilient farming. Our concerns for social justice should prevent exploitation regardless of age, gender, country, race, *and* species. Fortunately, these aims coincide: better farming means better housing and animal husbandry, local land stewardship, human health, social justice, and food security. And, while global concerns may eventually motivate reduced meat consumption, there are large areas of the world unsuitable for crop production, where the use of pastoral farming can assist good land management, and where veterinary science will hopefully focus more attention.

Increasingly, veterinary science will inform and become integrated with other areas of scientific research. As well as human medicine and ecology, it will combine with animal science, agronomics, nutritional science, business science, economics, sociology, anthropology, meteorology, and climatology. Veterinary science is part of our human effort to understand the world—to make it better (or at least to know how to cause less harm). It is through collaboration that we will achieve these aims.

Further reading

Chapter 1: All creatures great and small

A good book for animals in war is Gardiner's *The Animals' War* (Portrait Publishing, 2006). References for the history of veterinary and anthropic medicine include Cassidy et al.'s paper on 'Animal Roles and Traces in the History of Medicine', in *BJHS Themes* (2017, 1–23); Wilkinson's *Animals and Disease: An Introduction to the History of Comparative Medicine* (Cambridge University Press, 1992); and Rupke's *Vivisection in Historical Perspective* (Routledge, 1990). Fraser's *Understanding Animal Welfare* (UFAW/Wiley-Blackwell, 2008) provides an oversight of animal welfare as a concept. The famous novel by James Herriot is *All Creatures Great and Small*, now published by Pan. The oath is based on the one used in Kerala and is common across India, and based on a common format (with minor variations) used in other countries such as the USA, Canada, Kenya, Iran, the Philippines, and Sri Lanka. The Salihotra manuscript on the care and riding of horses is available at <https://commons.wikimedia.org/w/index.php?curid=12515260t>. One of Ashoka's pillars can be seen at <https://commons.wikimedia.org/wiki/File:Ashoka's_Pillar,_Vaishali.jpg>.

Chapter 2: Our families and other animals

The chapter title 'Our families and other animals' is a reference to Gerald Durrell's book *My Family and Other Animals*. Standard veterinary textbooks include Dyce, Sack, and Wensing's *Textbook of Veterinary Anatomy* (Saunders, 2017); Cunningham's *Textbook of Veterinary Physiology* (Saunders, 2010); Quinn et al.'s *Veterinary Microbiology and Microbial Disease* (Wiley-Blackwell, 2011); Mehlhorn's *Animal Parasites: Diagnosis, Treatment, Prevention* (Springer, 2016); Day and Schultz's *Veterinary Immunology: Principles and Practice* (C&C Press, 2014); and Zachary's *Pathologic Basis of Veterinary Disease* (Elsevier, 2016). Further consideration of animal welfare as a science is given in Mellor et al.'s *The Sciences of Animal Welfare* (UFAW/Wiley-Blackwell, 2009). A readable academic paper on the *Euhaplorchis californiensis* activity is Shaw et al.'s 'Parasite Manipulation of Brain Monoamines in California Killifish (Fundulus Parvipinnis) by the Trematode Euhaplorchis Californiensis', *Proceedings of the Royal Society of London B: Biological Sciences* 276(1659), 1137–46 (2009). Other lovely references in the OUP Very Short Introduction series are in Holland's *The Animal Kingdom* (2011); Wyatt's *Animal Behaviour* (2017); O'Shea's *The Brain* (2005); Evans's *Emotion* (2003); Allen's *The Cell* (2011); Slack's *Genes* (2014); Money's *Microbiology* (2014); Wayne and Bolker's *Infectious Diseases* (2015); Crawford's *Viruses* (2011); Amyes's *Bacteria* (2013); and James's *Cancer* (2011).

Chapter 3: Making illnesses better

There are of course many good textbooks on veterinary treatment for students and practitioners, and it would foolish to list them all. Particularly accessible references for veterinary decision-making and treatment include Aspinall's *Complete Textbook of Veterinary Nursing* (Elsevier, 2016); Girling's *Veterinary Nursing of Exotic Pets* (Wiley-Blackwell, 2013); Botzler and Brown's *Foundations of Wildlife Diseases* (University of California Press, 2014); and my *Animal Welfare in Veterinary Practice* (UFAW/Wiley, 2013). Pages for non-veterinarians on various diseases can be found on the Merck Veterinary Manual site at <http://www.msdvetmanual.com/en-gb/>. Further nice references in the OUP Very Short

Introduction series include Iversen's *Drugs* (2001); O'Donnell's *Anaesthesia* (2012); Bender's *Nutrition* (2012); and Boddice's *Pain* (2017).

Chapter 4: Making lives better

The saying 'Prevention is better than cure' is often attributed to Erasmus. Benjamin Franklin is also quoted as saying 'An ounce of prevention is worth a pound of cure', which appeared in the 4 February 1935 edition of the *Pennsylvania Gazette* (in which Benjamin Franklin did not use his own name, using instead the pseudonym 'An old citizen'). References on preventive work include Gudding et al.'s *Fish Vaccination* (Wiley Blackwell, 2014); Felippe's *Equine Clinical Immunology* (Wiley Blackwell, 2016); Hosey's *Zoo Animals: Behaviour, Management and Welfare* (OUP, 2013); Thrusfield's *Veterinary Epidemiology* (Blackwell, 2007); Pfeiffer's *Veterinary Epidemiology: An Introduction* (Wiley-Blackwell, 2009); and Hudson et al.'s *The Ecology of Wildlife Diseases* (OUP, 2002). A review of the discussion on tail docking is provided in Sutherland and Tucker's paper on 'The Long and Short of It: A Review of Tail Docking in Farm Animals', *Applied Animal Behaviour Science* 135(3): 179–91 (2011).

Chapter 5: Diseases across species

References on disease interactions across species include Atlas and Maloy's *One Health* (ASM Press, 2014); Zinsstag et al.'s *One Health: The Theory and Practice of Integrated Health Approaches* (CAB International, 2015); Palmer et al.'s *Oxford Textbook of Zoonoses: Biology, Clinical Practice, and Public Health Control* (OUP, 2013); Bauerfeind et al.'s *Zoonoses: Infectious Diseases Transmissible from Animals to Humans* (ASM Press, 2016); and Zinsstag et al.'s paper on 'From "One Medicine" to "One Health" and Systemic Approaches to Health and Well-being', in *Preventive Veterinary Medicine* I(101): 148–56 (2011). A more specific discussion of avian influenza is found in Bahl et al.'s paper on 'Ecosystem Interactions Underlie the Spread of Avian Influenza A Viruses with Pandemic Potential', *PLoS Pathogens* 12(5), e1005620 (2016). My thanks to Owen's mother for permission to use the image of him and Haatchi.

Chapter 6: Global veterinary medicine

Links between environmental and health concerns can be found in Brito et al.'s paper on 'Ill Nature: Disease Hotspots as Threats to Biodiversity', in the *Journal for Nature Conservation* 20(2): 72–5 (2012); Pongsiri et al.'s 'Biodiversity Loss Affects Global Disease Ecology', in *Bioscience* 59(11): 945–54 (2009); Jones et al.'s on 'Global Trends in Emerging Infectious Diseases', in *Nature* 451: 990–3 (2008); and Patz et al.'s on 'Unhealthy Landscapes: Policy Recommendations on Land Use Change and Infectious Disease Emergence', in *Environmental Health Perspectives* 112: 1092–8 (2004). Some specific points are described in more detail within Gillespie and Chapman's 'Prediction of Parasite Infection Dynamics in Primate Metapopulations based on Attributes of Forest Fragmentation', in *Conservation Biology* 20: 441–8 (2006); Riley et al., 'Exposure to Feline and Canine Pathogens in Bobcat and Gray Foxes in Urban and Rural Zones of a National Park in California', in the *Journal of Wildlife Diseases* 40: 11–22 (2004); and Walsh et al.'s 'Deforestation: Effects on Vector-borne Diseases', in *Parasitology* 106: S55–75 (1993). Links between disease, economics, and trade include Perry et al.'s *Investing in Animal Health Research to Alleviate Poverty* (ILRO, 2002); Brown and Gilfoyle's *Healing the Herds: Disease, Livestock Economies, and the Globalization of Veterinary Medicine* (Ohio University Press, 2010); Sherman's *Tending Animals in the Global Village: A Guide to International Veterinary Medicine* (Wiley, 2011); Smith and Kelly's *Food Security in a Global Economy: Veterinary Medicine and Public Health* (University of Pennsylvania Press, 2008); and the forthcoming book by D'Silva and Webster on *The Meat Crisis* (Routledge, 2017). The International Livestock Research Institute highlights geographic links in their *Mapping of Poverty and Likely Zoonoses Hotspots*, which can be found at <https://www.ilri.org/node/1244>.

Index

Index

SOCIAL MEDIA
Very Short Introduction

Join our community

www.oup.com/vsi

- Join us online at the official Very Short Introductions **Facebook** page.
- Access the thoughts and musings of our authors with our online **blog**.
- Sign up for our monthly **e-newsletter** to receive information on all new titles publishing that month.
- Browse the full range of Very Short Introductions online.
- Read **extracts** from the Introductions for free.
- If you are a teacher or lecturer you can order inspection copies quickly and simply via our website.